THE HIDDEN AGENDA

Dr. David Sneed
and
Dr. Sharon Sneed

A
JANET
THOMA
BOOK

THOMAS NELSON PUBLISHERS
Nashville

Copyright © 1991 by Dr. David Sneed and Dr. Sharon Sneed

All rights reserved. Written permission must be secured from the publisher to use or reproduce any part of this book, except for brief quotations in critical reviews or articles.

Published in Nashville, Tennessee, by Thomas Nelson, Inc., and distributed in Canada by Lawson Falle, Ltd., Cambridge, Ontario.

Scripture quotations are from the NEW KING JAMES VERSION of the Bible. Copyright © 1979, 1980, 1982, Thomas Nelson, Inc., Publishers.

Library of Congress Cataloging-in-Publication Data

Sneed, David, 1953–
    The hidden agenda / David Sneed and Sharon Sneed.
      p.   cm.
    "A Janet Thoma book."
    Includes bibliographical references.
    ISBN 0-8407-7491-5 (pbk.)
    1. Alternative medicine. 2. New Age movement—Controversial literature. 3. Quacks and quackery. 4. Medical misconceptions.
I. Sneed, Sharon, 1953–   II. Title.
R733.S64   1991
615.8'56—dc20   91–35748
                                            CIP

Printed in the United States of America

1 2 3 4 5 6 7 — 96 95 94 93 92

CONTENTS

ACKNOWLEDGMENTS

The support and interest of many people were instrumental in the development and writing of this book. Among these, special encouragement came from Joe and Patty Flack, Nell and Don Sunukjian, and Gay and Shannon Cox. We also appreciate the support of Winn Chapman and Bruce Hurt, M.D.

Special thanks goes to Texe and Wanda Marrs for their insight and materials on the New Age Movement as well as documentary support from Living Truth Ministries of Austin. The staff and services of the Texas Medical Association Library in Austin provided essential medical literature for this complex subject.

Renee Barger and Janice Lyons of Asheville, North Carolina, provided invaluable material on the influence of alternative medicine within church organizations.

Many thanks to John Renner, M.D., and William Jarvis, Ph.D., who provided personal advice and whose organizations continue to address the issue of health fraud on a national level.

The expertise of Kay Strom, the fine editorial work of Janet Thoma and Susan Salmon, and the commitment of Thomas Nelson Publishing to this project have seen it through to completion. Our heartfelt thanks goes to these and others who have enabled our efforts.

INTRODUCTION

Desperation often breeds frantic ill-advised decisions. And nothing catapults us into these hopeless situations more effectively than severe health problems. We resist aging. We fight disease. We look for answers and cures when we have been told there are none, save prayer. All are noble efforts; and, in fact, we have written entire books on how to do just these things—prevent illness from occurring.

There is of late a new presence in healthcare which calls itself alternative or complementary medicine. It consists of legions of practitioners in a vast and varied network of alternative medicine who often have nothing more in common than a severe distrust and even antagonism toward scientific medical approaches. Its adherents preach about the power of universal energies, inner spirits and guides that can help to heal, and the fact that you can heal yourself—if only you try hard enough. Some claim ancient wisdom is the key while others clearly associate with the New Age movement and are anticipatory for the new world to come—one which they claim will be created out of man's own goodness and self-realization.

Some have well-appointed offices in the world's leading medical centers, are on the *New York Times* best-seller lists, and proudly display their M.D. diplomas on the walls. Others practice in obscure little places catering to the "socially conscious" and trendy people of the world. Many freely mix medicine and spirituality from an eclectic grab bag of world religions and arcane healing practices designed to appeal to the broadest possible audience.

There have always been healers proclaiming this same message of herbal remedies, spiritual healing guides, and a distrust of "Western" medicine. We recognize them as witch doctors, shamans, and medicine men who practice primitive healing methods in remote tribal areas of the world. Today the homeopath, the psychic healer, the alternative physician promoting visualization, acupuncture, crystal healing, iridology, reflexology, or many other methods of today's alternative medicine movement would have us embrace without question the unproven, unscientific methods and occult philosophies they espouse. The witch doctor has returned and seeks to change the practice of medicine forever.

David Sneed, D.O.
Sharon Sneed, Ph.D.

Chapter One

THE RETURN OF
THE WITCH DOCTOR

On a sunny afternoon in early spring, an attractive dark-haired woman in her mid-forties walked into our clinic here in Austin, Texas, where I practice family medicine and my wife, Sharon, a registered dietitian with her Ph.D., is a nutrition consultant.

The woman introduced herself as Pam. "I don't have an appointment," she told the receptionist, "but it's important that I see a doctor today. I don't mind waiting."

It was 4 P.M. before I was able to see Pam. Yet, when she sat down across the desk from me, she seemed in no hurry to get to the point of her visit. An articulate woman, she wanted to tell me about her incredible journey into the healing rituals of the alternative medicine movement. "I was a problem child," Pam admitted with a trace of a smile. Although she was raised in a churchgoing family, she emerged from her rebellious teenage years an avowed atheist. "It was just as well," she said. "Whenever I mentioned anything spiritual, my husband got angry. In fact he became more and more angry about everything, it seemed," Pam said. "I had trouble keeping our marriage together."

1

Pam and her husband eventually got a divorce, and she found herself raising two adolescent children alone. Depression drove her to seek counseling. Within months her new therapist opened the metaphysical door of alternative medicine to this vulnerable woman.

"My counselor listened to me," Pam said. "He really cared about my problems. He really cared about me. Finally someone had some answers." Pam's counselor was a member of the Baha'i World Faith, a non-Christian cult that broke off from fundamental Islam in Iran. Teaching the basic unity of all world religions, Baha'i emphasizes the equality of religious leaders such as Muhammad, Moses, Buddha, Krishna, Bahaullah, and Jesus Christ.

At the counselor's encouragement, Pam enrolled in a local metaphysical philosophy school. "I learned so much!" Pam proceeded to recount her indoctrination into the mystical experiences of past life regression, dream therapy, contacts with spirits, and Eastern meditation. I looked at this woman sitting in the chair across the desk from me. Shoulder length hair, an attractive business suit, tastefully applied makeup—she looked little different from a hundred other middle-aged women I've seen in my office. Certainly she didn't look like someone with one foot in the world of the occult.

"The school changed my life," Pam exclaimed. "I gave up my career as a music teacher. Now I'm a massage therapist."

I glanced up at the clock. It was getting late and I still had hospital rounds to do. "My nurse said it was important for you to see me today. What's the medical problem that brought you here?" I asked. "Oh, I don't have a medical problem," Pam insisted. "I see a homeopathic physician regularly. When Anne, my twelve-year-old daughter, had some problems, I took her to see a reflexologist who recommended that all three of us begin a macrobiotic diet, which we did. I'm fine, and so are Anne and Todd—he's my fourteen-year-old son."

I could not believe the woman's words. We had talked for more than thirty minutes now. She had waited to see me for an hour and a half. Yet she had no physical ailment? I decided to probe a little further.

"Macrobiotic diet? Did you know Zen Buddhism is behind the macrobiotic diet?" I asked.

"Really?" Pam exclaimed. "That's great! You know, I was a Buddhist three lives ago."

Pam explained that although she considered herself "first a Christian," since she was raised in a Presbyterian church, she was convinced that the teaching of Buddha and Muhammad were equally as valid as those of Jesus Christ.

"I think my Christianity comes from my encounter with a spirit guide," she said. "The spirit was Jesus himself. He told me so."

By now it was 5:30, yet I listened in fascination. I could not believe that this intelligent woman could mix Eastern religion and Christianity so easily.

Pam went on to tell me about an "energy column," which she claimed descended from the heart of the universe and went right through her body. "That's what lets my soul travel out of my body and go on mystical journeys while I sleep," she said.

"Aren't you afraid of the spiritual forces you might encounter?" I asked.

"Oh, no! I learned in the New Age church I attend that we don't have to fear the dark spirits." As tears welled up in her eyes and her voice shook with emotion Pam continued, "Satan, you know, is not so different from you and me. All he really wants is a reunion with God. I feel so sorry for him."

For the first time since she walked into my office, Pam was silent. So was I.

I decided to try to understand why she was there one last time. "Well, what *can* I do for you?"

"I need a prescription for birth control pills," she said. "By tonight."

I told her she would need a physical and some lab work before I could prescribe any medication.

"No examination," she insisted. "Just the prescription. I know what I need!"

When I said I couldn't do that, her face hardened and her entire demeanor changed. "Just like a doctor!" she muttered as she stalked out of my office.

Pam was one of my first encounters with a patient who had totally embraced New Age religion after being influenced by alternative health care practitioners who promoted these beliefs. Needless to say, I never saw Pam again. Yet I have often wondered what has become of her as I now recognize many other people who have been influenced just as she was.

ALTERNATIVE HEALTH PRACTICES

Alternative medicine is known, among other things, for its emphasis on a holistic approach to its patients—theoretically, the consideration of each person as a whole, with a complex interaction of body, mind, and spirit. And who wouldn't want to be treated in this way? The best-selling book *Love Hunger,* by Dr. Frank Minirth, Dr. Paul Meier, Dr. Robert Hemfelt, and Dr. Sharon Sneed, is meeting just such a need for thousands of people across the nation who are struggling against food addiction. Unfortunately, however, many people seeking holistic treatment are now falling under the influence of practitioners with highly questionable health information and methods—and with equally questionable spiritual and emotional "treatment."

These alternative health practices run the gamut from innocent, even scientifically proven beneficial techniques, such as biofeedback and natural foods, to outright occult practices, such as spirit guides and psychic surgeons. Yet whether innocent or occult, alternative health care is being sought out by millions of people throughout our country.

According to Dr. Victor Herbert, a professor of medicine at Mount Sinai School of Medicine, in New York, and a noted medical fraud investigator, an incredible 26 billion dollars is spent each year by gullible and often desperate people on unproven, unscientific, and downright dangerous treatments, prescriptions, and medical devices.

"There is no such thing as 'orthodox versus alternative' therapy," Dr. Herbert insists. "There is simply responsible therapy (therapy that works), irresponsible therapy (therapy that does not work), and experimental therapy. Direct harms from quackery have ranged from minor to death. Indirect harm is often death from a cancer which responsible therapy could have cured."[1]

What is just as disturbing, considering the magnitude of its influence, is the rapidly expanding and largely unregulated holistic health industry run by mail-order nutritionists, Rolfers, colonic hygienists, shamans, faith healers, herbalists, polarity therapists, reflexologists, naturopaths, homeopaths, and psychic surgeons. The National Council Against Health Fraud says:

> Health fraud and quackery have become socially acceptable. Politicians openly lobby on behalf of Laetrile, orthomolecular psychiatry, chelation for heart disease, and numerous other questionable methods. Some health professionals have abandoned the scientific rigor of their disciplines to promote a myriad of pseudosciences under the guise of holistic health. . . . Quacks rob us of our money, our dignity, our health, and our lives.[2]

For instance, a patient suffering from abdominal pain called the director of the Scottsdale Holistic Medical Center in Arizona, and seventy-year-old Dr. Gladys McGarey, M.D., told her what to do: Drink ginger tea and apply a castor oil pack to her abdomen. The woman's discomfort, as it turned out, was caused by appendicitis, and what she needed was emergency surgery.

In her forty years of medical practice, Dr. McGarey has regularly prescribed such remedies for abdominal distress. She admits it's not a traditional medical practice. "But," she insists, "we have found it works."

Not for this patient. She is suing Dr. McGarey.[3]

Since practitioners of alternative health care claim to treat the whole individual, they suggest by their very name that scientific medicine has somehow failed to treat the whole person. Perhaps this charge is easy to make in light of the increasing specialization of medicine and the sometimes impersonal care a person may receive.

What is holistic medicine? Simply put, it is medical treatment based on the recognition that each of us is a whole person made up of the interacting elements of body, mind and spirit. Not a bad concept, both for patient and for health practitioner. It was this very aspect of medicine that drew me toward a medical career in the first place. Yet it is the adulteration of this concept that now presses us to write this book.

We have no doubt but what every competent physician recognizes the interaction of body and mind. Which of us can help but notice the added physical problems that accompany increased emotional stress in our patients? Recognizing the spiritual interaction, however, varies from doctor to doctor, and to a large degree it depends on his or her own personal spirituality. It is here in the area of spirit that we must be very careful; many so-called alternative practices are heavily steeped in false spirituality, Eastern mysticism, and New Age thought.

And what about the term "alternative medicine," the term most often used to describe this entire group of questionable medical practices? Because this term is recognizable and in common usage, we will generally use it when we refer to the largely unscientific, unproven, and—regrettably—often unsafe health practices which typically fall outside of what is considered mainstream medical practice. From acupuncture and aromatherapy to shamanism, yoga, and Zen macrobiotics, alternative medical practices not only span the alphabet; they run the gamut from clever blending of fact and fancy to complete foolishness.

In this book we will explore various types of alternative medical treatments.

We have divided the various aspects of alternative medicine into the following categories: natural, mind-cure, energy manipulation, and supernatural. Given that alternative medicine claims to be beneficial for virtually every form of physical and emotional illness currently unknown to science, there will undoubtedly be some overlap among the categories. Natural methods are those practices that purport to heal by use of means that are not technological or man-made. These include vitamin and herbal therapies; manual therapies such as chiropractic, massage, and Rolfing; homeopathic medicine with its extremely diluted potions made from natural substances; and other treatments which rely principally upon natural healing medications and methods.

Mind-cure therapies are those based on a belief in the power of mind over sickness. "Think yourself well" and "meditate to that perfect ideal of health" are typical messages coming from the teachings of Christian Science, Transcendental Meditation, and Yoga. Mind over illness is for many the long sought panacea for all sickness, both physical and emotional. Medically accepted and proven techniques such as hypnosis and biofeedback fall within this group. Unfortunately, their legitimate use is being distorted by the alternative medicine movement.

Energy manipulation is the basis for many alternative healing practices often associated with the New Age movement and its quasi-religious aspects. Belief in a powerful universal energy in and through all things is at the heart of many Eastern religions as well as in all practices which seek to manipulate this energy: acupuncture, reflexology, iridology, applied kinesiology, therapeutic touch, and crystal healing. Alternative advocates such as Kristin Olsen in her *Encyclopedia of Alternative Health Care* see the "marriage of Western and Eastern medicines" as opening "new cultural and philosophical horizons." Extolling the virtues of these unproven therapies, she points out that "Many professional health care providers integrate Chinese or Indian medicine-based philosophy or Buddhist spiritual principles into a Western health approach."[4]

Supernatural therapies are those that clearly step outside the realm of normal human experience into the occult world of spirits, out-of-body experiences, communication with the dead, and magical healing. Natural cause-and-effect explanations for these methods do not exist—unless one considers fraud a cause. For most people, this area of alternative medicine elicits at least some apprehension. Yet today's alternative healers, if not able to convince you to see a shaman or witch doctor personally, will gladly introduce you to these same occult techniques through guided visualization and personal contact with a spirit guide of your own.

We have listed many of the alternative health practices in each of these four categories in the Appendix. Later in this book we will look at each of these practices individually to evaluate its effectiveness.

WHO LOOKS FOR ALTERNATIVE CARE?

What makes average, everyday, intelligent people like Pam seek such strange and questionable treatment? That very question was posed at a panel discussion at the 1988 National Health Fraud Conference at Kansas City, Missouri. According to Naomi Kulakow, officer of Consumer Affairs of the Food and Drug Association, three types of patients tend to seek out questionable treatments.

1. People Who Are Not Really Ill in the First Place

People who are not sick tend to look for prevention. They want to stay well, to be assured that their good health will continue. Scientific medicine can't give absolute assurance. When a patient goes to his doctor and says, "Prescribe some vitamins for me," a physician will look at the situation scientifically.

"You don't really need vitamins," he will likely say. "Just eat a balanced diet. That will give you all the vitamins you need. Read this book on how to eat a healthy diet—and don't forget to do some aerobic exercise four times a week."

That seems to be a satisfactory answer to me. But what if this isn't what the patient wanted to hear? He wants a quick fix as well as an outright promise of good health. He wants a secret, an inside track. So he starts listening to the advertising for bogus health aids and nutritional supplements. There, he does hear secrets and learns of inside tracks. In fact, he gets fantastic promises and unconditional guarantees. Whatever he wants to hear, someone is ready to tell him. Whatever he's willing to buy, someone is ready to sell.

Charismatic leaders and convincing proponents of a certain method often have a great deal of influence. Although they give little information about what a patient will actually be getting for her money, she willingly writes the checks in hopes of getting those remarkable results she hears promised. She doesn't see that what she actually gets is at best highly questionable.

"Never did I think I would consider something as disgusting as coffee enemas," says Eugene, a college instructor. "Yet there I was, listening to the 'doctor's' spiel, my checkbook in my hand."

"Balancing bottles of vitamins on my outstretched arms? What kind of diagnosis is that?" says Carolyn. "Yet, there I was. And I paid for all the stuff he prescribed. Maybe I felt intimidated."

The search for alternative methods often allows people to reassert some control over their situation. This feels good. It's a great antidote for a frustrating sense of helplessness.

Patients today are far more medically sophisticated and aware than they have ever been before. Yet at the same time their trust in the authority of physicians has greatly decreased. Alternative therapists see this, and they are ready to step in to fill the gap. Their message: "Traditional doctors don't understand. We do."

Like Pam, most people who are deeply involved in alternative healing don't jump right in. They take one small step, perhaps just an inquisitive one. At first they may step back from a practice and say, "It's sort of weird." They may even add, "I can't believe real people get involved in that." Then, step by step, they go deeper and deeper until they are hooked.

Evelyn is a good example of someone who began by dabbling. A quiet, slender young woman of twenty-six, Evelyn
came to see me about her depression. As we talked, I noticed
she was wearing a crystal obelisk pendant around her neck.

"Why are you wearing the crystal?" I asked.

Evelyn told me her boss had recognized her depression and
recommended she take a "light-weavers course and get rejuve-
nated." This eight week metaphysical course—sort of a New
Age healing sampler—served as an introduction to such practices as meditation, past life regression, crystal healing, and
channeling.

"They did this rock thing where we sat in a circle with rocks
and crystals around us. We were supposed to feel the vibrations. Then they taught us to meditate, to do past life regres-
sions, and even to make contact with a spirit guide."

"What did you think about all that?" I asked.

"Kind of silly," Evelyn said. "I mean, some of it was pretty
far out." Then she quickly added, "But there were a lot of good
points about it, too. It filled a need for me. It made me feel
better about myself."

"Do you think your crystal has any power?"

"No," Evelyn said. "I just like it because it's so pretty."

Maybe so. But Evelyn now regularly practices guided meditation. She tells me she has even tried to contact a spirit guide.

"It's not a spiritual thing," she insists. "All that metaphysical
stuff is just interesting."

As Evelyn's case shows, alternative medicine can allow the
freedom to pick and choose. Some of it may be appealing,
while other aspects may move too flagrantly in one direction or
another. For instance, someone might not be willing to become
involved immediately with communicating with a spirit guide,
yet that person may be happy to have his "universal energy"
manipulated by a practitioner doing therapeutic touch.

2. Those with Chronic Pain

It's not hard to understand how patients suffering from
chronic pain can be sucked in by charlatan practitioners. Often

such patients have psychological problems that go along with the pain—conditions such as depression and stress. These need to be treated, too. If the physician doesn't recognize the psychological source of his patient's discomfort and simply tells her, "It's nothing" or "It's all in your mind," he is running the risk of driving that patient right into the arms of the quacks. What the suffering patient wants is an answer. If her physician can't give it to her, she determines to seek out someone who can.

Many people who are subjected to health food store promotions, raving friends and relatives, even religious teachings, never really question the testimonials they hear. It sounds good, they reason. It evidently worked for someone. "Leave no stone unturned," they are told. "Why not give it a try?" Dramatic stories of miraculous cures are told and retold to them. They are given books to read. They are drawn deeper and deeper into an involvement with unproven, even suspicious, practices. Without realizing what has happened, people find themselves lured into the most unlikely health care systems.

3. Those with a Terminal Illness

Probably the saddest victims of all are those with a terminal illness such as cancer or AIDS. In their eyes, scientific medicine has nothing more to offer them. They may feel abandoned and hopeless. Why not look to someone who claims to have an answer? Even an empty promise may seem better than no hope at all.

"My counselor listened to me," Pam had told me. "He really cared about my problems. He really cared about me."

You say you would never be so gullible? You say you would never fall for such unscientific practices? Don't be so sure. The fact is, under the duress of a serious illness, any of us might seek alternative therapy—especially when it is a treatment recommended by friends or family, or when it has been published in a best-selling book.

Sometimes the patient's own physician points the way. "Have you ever thought about meditating?" the doctor asks. Or maybe it's simply that a person has a preference for things natural. "Herbs, potions—this is all natural medicine," she reasons. "It has to be good for me."

DOES ALTERNATIVE MEDICINE REALLY HEAL?

You may ask, "Do these methods work or don't they?" Good question. Let's approach the answer scientifically. When medical science asks, "Does it work or doesn't it?" it quickly follows with another question: "Can you *prove* it works?" But where most types of alternative health care are involved, proven methods aren't part of the program. Instead, practitioners simply offer anecdotal stories or pseudo-scientific studies published in bogus journals.

"This patient had cancer, and he got well because he meditated," we are enthusiastically informed. Now, it may be that this patient was also undergoing chemotherapy and radiation therapy, but that's not mentioned. All that's talked about is the meditation.

"The diet cured my cancer," a healthy looking man may announce. The fellow may have died of cancer the year after he made his victorious claim, but that little detail isn't mentioned, either.

"I look ten years younger after using this treatment," a smiling woman may tell us. Or "I lost thirty pounds in just three weeks." Since we never saw the woman before, we have no proof but her word—and possibly a picture she selected to show us.

On the other hand, there are numerous documented cases of alternative medical practices which have led not only to harm, but to the death of patients. Even though Pam, the young woman we met at the beginning of this chapter, did not seem to have been harmed by her journey into unproven and ineffectual alternative health practices, both she and her children are at great risk should they become seriously ill. The literature is filled with instances of just such misguided tragedies.

Seventeen-month-old Lorie Atikian died from malnutrition and pneumonia. Just eight months before, she was a perfectly healthy baby. By the time she died, little Lorie had lost almost all her hair, had a terrible skin condition, and was so emaciated that the paramedics who arrived at her home thought they were being given a doll to treat.

Lorie's parents loved her. Concerned about modern food additives, pesticide residues, and drugs, they consulted a local herbologist to advise them. By herbology standards, this man was qualified to practice. He had learned his trade in Germany through studying books, and had obtained a mail order doctoral degree in Naturopathy from Bernadean University in Las Vegas, Nevada.

Armed with his books and his bogus "degree," this herbologist/naturopath operated two herbal stores, gave seminars on herbal medicine, and had written a book which described how to heal diabetes, epilepsy, tuberculosis, tumors, and paralysis—all by "touchless massage."

Before Lorie was born, her mother, anxious to do right by her family, took a course in herbology and healing from this man. He convinced her to "remain pure" for the sake of the child she was carrying. If she did so, he promised, the child would become a "super baby."

What he advocated was an organic, vegetarian diet. To help her along, he sold her a special juicer for $400. (They already had a juicer, but theirs, he said, "burned the nutrition" right out of the fruits and vegetables.)

When baby Lorie became ill, she was treated with royal jelly, homeopathic medicine, and an herbal brew, concocted by the naturopath. He also treated the baby with electromagnetic vitalizing machines, which were supposed to stimulate her blood. They even had attachments, such as an electrified comb which was supposed to liven up her hair. Take her to the doctor? Oh, no, they were told. That would be like "holding a loaded gun to Lorie's head and pulling the trigger."

After little Lorie died, her parents were charged with child neglect and were found guilty. Their real crime was that they believed this quack practitioner.

IS WHATEVER WORKS ALL RIGHT?

Practitioners in the holistic field tend to take an entirely different tack than do traditional physicians. "Anything and everything we do is okay," they insist. "Whatever works for you is all right." Does that advice really make sense?

If you're going to a physician for advice, you don't want to hear, "Well, sure, go ahead and do whatever you're doing. If it works for you, it's okay." That's not really advice at all. A physician who says such things is just acting as a cheerleader. He's merely encouraging you. Anybody can do that. The reason you go to a physician is because you want advice on what to do and what not to do based on sound medical facts.

Pam seemed physically healthy. Unfortunately other people are not so lucky.

Toxic side effects and even deaths are well documented as the direct result of several so-called alternative therapies. Even claims of improved "quality of life" in alternative patients have become extremely doubtful since the findings published in the *New England Journal of Medicine,* April 1991. Two groups of patients with extensive cancer and a predicted survival of less than one year were studied. One group received conventional medical cancer treatments, including chemotherapy and radiation. The other group was treated at a famous "alternative" clinic in California with an unproven "immune-enhancing" vaccine, vegetarian diets, and coffee enemas. At the end of the study, neither group had a significantly improved survival rate. Yet there was a difference. The conventional treatment group reported a much better quality of life during their few remaining months. Not only are the alternative treatments ineffective; they aren't even as user-friendly as most people think.

ARE ALL ALTERNATIVES HARMFUL?

So, are all alternatives to traditional healing methods bad? Not at all. In fact, some may consider me an alternative health practitioner, since I'm an osteopathic physician.

Osteopathic physicians are one of two groups of fully licensed physicians in the United States. Medical doctors (M.D.s) make up about 95 percent of all this country's fully licensed physicians. The rest are osteopathic doctors (D.O.s). The difference between the two? There is a push within the osteopathic schools to "teach more holistically." What this means is that we osteopathic physicians recognize the interrelationship of various bodily systems within the human being. We aim toward looking at an individual as a whole person and receive additional training in the treatment of musculo-skeletal disorders.

You say this sounds very much like what the alternative health care movement does in their integration of body, mind, and spirit? Not quite.

Osteopathic physicians, while practicing holistically, have embraced rather than flaunted medical science. We concentrate on the bodily systems, on the emotional aspects, and upon scientific concepts of disease.

Perhaps I am so interested in a book such as this because I can somewhat relate to these alternative health practitioners. I know what it's like to be a minority in the medical field. I understand the necessity of at times having to stand up and speak with authority for the practices I have learned and the skills I've acquired. I know what it feels like to have to explain myself and to have to be extra scrupulous about what I do. I know what it is to be called upon to justify myself and my practices because I'm not a "regular medical doctor."

And yet there are distinct and important differences between most osteopathic doctors and the alternative health care practitioners. For the most part, osteopathic physicians are relegated to the scientific medical/physical side of things rather than to the alternative health care side, since we are fully licensed in all fifty states to prescribe medication and to perform surgery. We can, in fact, practice in any area of medicine, from neurosurgery to pediatric care, from psychiatry to sports medicine.

I myself am a family physician. I'm residency trained and licensed to practice medicine and surgery in the state of Texas. I have hospital privileges and take care of patients of all ages, from newborns to senior citizens in nursing homes. The only difference between me and my M.D. partner is that during my medical school I had some additional hours of training in manipulative medicine—that is, the manual treatment of musculo-skeletal problems.

This is an adjunct to my therapy. I now primarily use it with patients who suffer from low back strain, whiplash injuries, stiff necks, or other such problems. I do not claim to dissolve gallstones with it, nor do I try to cure diabetes. Certainly I don't believe such problems as thyroid disease or multiple sclerosis or cancer or AIDS can be better treated with manipulation.

One of the major distinctions of osteopathic physicians is that they have been willing to grow—to learn as they have been presented with an ever-growing body of scientific knowledge and research. As effective antibiotics and other medications have been developed, osteopathic physicians have incorporated them into their treatment programs. We enthusiastically embrace effective, modern surgical techniques and modern medical care. Our training in manipulation, which we use to help with musculo-skeletal problems, simply gives osteopathic physicians an additional tool in the fight against disease.

Unfortunately, growing numbers of misguided doctors, osteopaths and M.D.s, are incorporating New Age health concepts into their practice. Many of the practices we will discuss have the identical philosophical background to that touted by the New Age religious movement. And certain methods and techniques, such as crystal therapy and channeling, are part and parcel of the New Age movement itself.

New Age medicine has become a growth industry. Kevin

Baadsgaard, director of marketing for Nature's Sunshine Products, the largest capsule makers of dehydrated herbs in the country, reports that business is booming for the natural health food industry (vitamins, herbs, minerals). It is expanding by 15 to 20 percent a year.

Here in Austin, Texas, a local New Age bookstore (non-profit, tax-exempt) reported to the *Austin Business Journal* gross sales climbing over a three-year period from $50,000 to over $300,000 annually. This same publication reported over 600 New Age related businesses now operating here in the capital city of Texas.

Any alternative health care practice that has embraced New Age philosophy may not only be physically and emotionally damaging to patients, but spiritually damaging. Doctors are not against alternative health care in general, but only the unproven and unsafe methods. We are also concerned about and caution against those practices that have blended with New Age religious philosophy.

In the next two chapters we will look at the potential harm these practices pose to unwary patients. Then in chapter 4 we offer you a standard by which to evaluate them—thirteen red flags to watch for as you consider any alternative health care practice.

In the second part of this book we will look at the alternative health care methods in each category, and expose the myths that often creep into this kind of care. For example, in chapter 5 we will examine many people's assumption that a natural product has to be better. Many are willing to lay down their money for their conviction. But does natural always mean better? Does natural guarantee safety? There are those who claim it does. Naturopathy, homeopathy, chiropractic, massage therapy, macrobiotics, herbalism—all are, or they all claim to be, totally natural. But which will heal and which will harm? It's not as easy to determine as many think, as you'll see.

Does mind over matter really work? Can we truly think ourselves well? Christian Science says so. It's what they don't say that is frightening. What is Transcendental Meditation? How about yoga? Are hypnosis and biofeedback legitimate medical practices? The answers we give in chapter 6, "Can You Think Yourself Well?" might surprise you.

Is there such a thing as universal energy? If so, how can it be harnessed and used for our healing and well-being? Energy manipulative therapies range from acupuncture and therapeutic touch to crystals and iridology (a so-called science based on "reading" the irises of the eyes). Some pretty strange stuff here; we'll talk about that in chapter 7, which looks at the myth, "May the Force Be with You."

And what about those therapies that rely on the downright supernatural? In chapter 8, "Communicating with the Spirits," we will look at the out-and-out occultic practices that underlie and pervade the alternative health care system. From a resurgence of the practices of ancient witch doctors and channeling for spirit guides to psychic surgery, such practices are surprisingly widespread.

In chapter 9, "Anything That Works Is Okay," we will consider the last myth: As long as a product works, it is okay to use or prescribe it. Should doctors prescribe placebos for their patients? Is this lying to the patient, or are placebos a legitimate alternative to prescription medicine?

Finally, in chapter 10, "Where Do We Go from Here?" we will look at the superstars of the alternative health care movement to help you evaluate these best-selling authors and well-known practitioners.

We Americans are notorious for our do-something, do-anything, even-if-it's-the-wrong-thing-it's-better-than-nothing approach to problem solving. It's true in our quest for health as well as in other areas of our life. Take control. Be aggressive. Be optimistic. You can win the battle. These are our prevailing attitudes. For many of us, it's often just too hard to accept the fact that there is such a thing as incurable disease.

If you are to be a wise and healthy person, it's not enough simply to know the practices out there. Should the time come for you or someone you care about to make a choice—and that time will come to nearly all of us—you will need more than background information. You will need specific guidelines. How else are you to choose wisely and well?

Without a doubt, whether or not a specific therapy works will be an important concern. But perhaps there is an even greater concern for Christians: the spiritual implications of a specific therapy. When we look at Pam's story, we can clearly see that alternative medicine and so-called holistic healers can easily become stepping stones that lead to a world of spiritual deception. The witch doctor is back in business, and he is hard at work. His "patients" include your friends and neighbors, maybe even your family members. You may even be one yourself.

How can you know what is dangerous? How can you determine where the spiritual snares lie? How can you identify the deceivers? Answering such questions is the purpose of this book. Join us as we explore the world of alternative medicine.

Chapter Two

WHAT DOES IT HURT?
Exposing Potential Dangers

A person who is faced with a serious illness lives on an emotional roller coaster. There are the dizzying ups and downs. The threat of death and the exhilaration of a possible cure. All the twists and turns, the long uphill climbs and the hopeful heights of remission. No one expressed this death-defying ride better than comedienne Gilda Radner in her autobiography, *It's Always Something*. The book chronicles her intense efforts to find a cure for her illness and her subsequent journey into the world of alternative medicine.

"I was tired, in pain and running low-grade fevers," Gilda wrote. "I was on too much medication. I decided to see an acupuncturist because friends had begun to suggest alternatives to my medical care."[1] When her doctors were unable to correctly diagnose Gilda's disease, she decided to see an acupuncturist. He did his work, but her stomach began to swell, and she continued to lose weight.

A well-meaning friend gave Gilda the name of a "doctor of holistic medicine." "The doctor used a technique developed in Germany," Gilda wrote. "He placed some metal device on pulse points in my body."[2] He then prescribed herbal preparations and coffee enemas, plus vitamins and minerals he said were missing in Gilda's body. She said she had what seemed like hundreds of pills and bottles, holistic drops, bags of seeds and leaves, and cans of food supplements—all accompanied by rigorous schedules of when to take them and what to do.

Gilda Radner was an intelligent lady who certainly could afford the best of specialists. So why was she submitting to pins in her ears and coffee enemas? She answers that the holistic doctor paid attention to her, calling her every day, asking her how she felt and what was going on, changing this or that if it didn't seem to be working. At least, she thought, the doctor took her seriously.

The thought behind all this seems to be: Alternative medicine can't hurt, and it just might be the answer.

WHAT ARE THE DANGERS?

One of the most dangerous myths surrounding alternative medical care is that it may help, and if it doesn't, at least it won't hurt. The truth is, alternative practices seldom help, and they certainly can hurt. We see eight possible dangers of alternative health care treatment: failure to diagnose, failure to treat, emotional harm, wasted money, physical threats, toxic effects, diverted resources, and loss of reality.

1. Failure to Diagnose

Many alternative healing systems rely upon such questionable methods as reading the irises of your eyes, palm reading, aura diagnosis, and therapeutic touch diagnosis. Some of their methods, such as pendulum diagnoses and diagnoses made through a spirit guide, are outright occultic.

If a practitioner can convince you there's nothing wrong with you that he can't cure, you aren't likely to seek out medical techniques that really might help. The time you lose could cost you your life.

Dr. Victor Herbert, professor of medicine at Mount Sinai School of Medicine and noted medical fraud investigator, writes:

> Quacks are health robbers. Dripping charisma, pity and charm, they rob cancer patients of their money, their health and their lives. They are the cruelest killers, and most importantly they rob patients of their time. The time patients spend with quacks gives the cancer time to spread so that proper treatment is delayed to a time when the cancer is so widespread that proper treatment is powerless to stop the inexorable course to death.[5]

Fortunately, Gilda Radner hadn't given up seeing her internist. Yet this presented another problem: "Do I tell the doctors about each other? East meets West in Gilda's body. Western medicine down my throat, Eastern medicine up my butt." She chose to stay quiet.

On October 20, 1986, Gilda got a call from her internist. It seemed her bloodwork had shown up an irregularity in her liver function test.

"What does it mean?" she screeched into the phone.

The doctor would have to recheck it. That's all he'd say.

It was Monday, and the doctor wasn't going to see Gilda until Thursday. So early Tuesday morning she went to see her holistic doctor, who put her on a special powdered protein diet.

By Thursday, Gilda was in such bad shape her internist admitted her to the hospital. "At last someone believes me," she wrote. "At last someone will find out what's wrong."

It was while she was in the hospital that her internist told her, "We've discovered a malignancy." Gilda had ovarian cancer. She was absolutely devastated.

Yet with typical good humor, she wrote in her book: "Suddenly I had to spend all my time getting well. I was fighting for my life against cancer, a more lethal foe than even the interior decorator."

2. Failure to Treat

Hand in hand with a failure to diagnose goes a failure to treat. If no one knows what's wrong, how can the problem be effectively treated?

Many of the methods in the alternative health care system take what we call a "shotgun approach" to treatment. Energy manipulation systems are good examples. They seek to align and balance energy fields in a nonspecific way even when the problems may be something such as an acute infection or depression that could and should be treated specifically. Without proper diagnosis, there can be no real treatment. Failure to treat a little boy with meningitis will result in his death. Failure to treat a young girl with bone cancer will end in her death. Failure to treat a woman with breast cancer will end in her death. (Specific documented cases of death from these diseases because of a failure to treat are given in chapter 6.)

Failure to treat constitutes malpractice on the broadest scale. Consider the "Revici method," one of the quack remedies for cancer listed by the Unproven Methods Committee of the American Cancer Society. After a thorough investigation, this mixture of oils and selenium—a true snake-oil if there ever was one—was pronounced worthless. Yet Revici continued to use it to treat cancer patients.

One patient was "treated" for fourteen months, long enough for her breast cancer to spread so widely it required massive medical surgery, chemotherapy, and radiation. When this former patient brought a suit against Revici, he claimed in his defense that he had told the woman to have a lumpectomy. And he pointed out that she had signed an informed consent agreeing to take his treatment. The jury was unimpressed. The woman was awarded 1 million dollars.[4]

Yet even though lawsuits have been brought against such practitioners, and even though judgments have been rendered against them, the practices continue. Revici has been selling his product in the state of New York for thirty years. Since most alternative health care workers are not licensed, no one can put them out of business by revoking their licenses. For some patients, the failure to treat may result in death. No one knows how many patients have died because they went to Revici and others like him, instead of to competent physicians for treatment.

3. Emotional Harm

After her first surgery, Gilda Radner was certain her cancer was gone. Nine courses of chemotherapy were prescribed by an oncologist, who also suggested relaxation therapy. The psychotherapist who helped with this introduced Gilda to the Wellness Clinic, "a place people could fight for recovery along with their physicians."

This wellness clinic was very much a part of the medical community in Los Angeles. One of the things taught about fighting cancer was that the first line of defense is the person's immune system. There was a great deal of emphasis on strengthening the immune system through visualization, imagery, nutrition, and the like.

From that point on, the clinic was to be a vital part of Gilda's life. She learned to make the treatment work for her both physically and psychologically. She learned to use techniques of visualization and relaxation to imagine she was helping the chemicals fight the cancer cells.

The Wellness Clinic group sessions of visualization and relaxation and the sharing that went on with other cancer patients were helpful to Gilda. There was an ever present optimism within the group. If statistics indicated that only 8 percent survive a particular cancer, the group affirmed that every one of them had just as much right to be in that 8 percent as anybody else. Group members urged each other to do everything possible to fight their cancer—anything to participate in the recovery process.

Any technique or therapy in which anyone wanted to be involved was acceptable at the clinic. If a person felt something had been helpful, then it was okay. Yet Gilda wrote about one woman whose story had a deep effect on her:

> She was diagnosed with a particular kind of lymphoma. She immediately went everywhere for every possible cure other than the recognized medical one. She went to Mexico. She went to Europe. She did all the spiritual, mystical cures. She spent thousands and thousands of dollars traveling, looking for an answer. After a year of doing this she had some side effects from experimental treatment that were even worse than her cancer. They drove her back to her medical doctor, and he put her on chemotherapy. She had to take these big pills . . . and started to feel better, and her lymphoma was under control.[5]

At the Wellness Clinic, Gilda was told that death is a part of life. She couldn't accept this.

Gilda was determined to cover all bases. Before her "second look" surgery, she bought an amethyst crystal to wear on a chain around her neck. The surgery went well and there were no obvious signs of cancer. Multiple biopsies were done. Out of forty-two biopsies, only two microscopic cancer cells were found, and they weren't highly active. Nevertheless, those two cells were malignant. The doctor suggested six additional chemotherapies. Gilda was terribly upset. She thought the chemotherapy was behind her. Her hair was growing back. Panic set in. Believing that unless she took drastic measures the cancer was going to kill her, she determined to work harder, to meditate twice a day, to be more positive.

After she finished her second round of chemotherapy, it was recommended that Gilda have radiation therapy.

"Just because of two little microscopic cells?" she asked. The doctor insisted it was better to get rid of it all, and to do it now. The wellness community encouraged her to go along with the program. As for Gilda, she was still trying to hedge her bets: She went to her radiation treatments but also brought her crystal with her every day.

By Christmas 1987, Gilda was finished with her treatments and there was a great celebration. She was even featured on the cover of *Life* magazine. It was only when she read the accompanying article that she discovered there was just a 30 percent chance of surviving ovarian cancer and that she wouldn't know for at least a year and a half whether she was really in remission. No one had ever told her that. She had been allowed to think her ordeal was over.

Three months later, Gilda moved to Connecticut. Knowing she had to get some blood work done, Gilda looked over the names of Connecticut oncologists in the telephone book and called one who was nearby. "If I complained of any pain or discomfort, this Connecticut oncologist would mention that it could be the cancer," Gilda wrote. "I didn't like him: he was gruff and impatient."[6]

In time, Gilda was called in by the new doctor she didn't even like and told, "There is a problem."

Her positive, wellness-community world fell apart, but she continued to fight. She now used her visualizations not just for relaxation but as a mental means of fighting the cancer. She imagined battles going on inside her, with armored horsemen killing the cancer cells. She made the pictures as graphic and clear as possible, determined to win.

The Fallacy of the Patient's Will

In the realm of the alternative health movement, we see again and again how the responsibility for the disease is placed squarely on the shoulders of the suffering person. This is also true of some "Christian" approaches. Monte Kline, a popular Christian health writer, authored a book entitled *God's Plan for Your Body* in which he affirmed this:

> When you wake up some day and find out you have cancer or heart disease or arthritis, or you have M.S., or whatever it is, you shouldn't wonder what caused this. You see, you did it. You did it in not being conformed to Christ's Lordship, the Lordship of His creation and the way he made things to function.[7]

Barbara Sigmund was mayor of Princeton, New Jersey, when a medical exam revealed she had eye cancer and that it had spread to various parts of her body. "Very soon thereafter, the self-help books started arriving," she reported. "I had caused my own cancer, they told me, so it was up to me to cure it."[8]

Having to accept such responsibility leads only to a great deal of guilt and self-recrimination. The burden is doubled when, regardless of what they try, patients don't get well. As a patient feels more and more guilty about his personal responsibility for his illness, he may sink deeper and deeper into depression. He may withdraw from all treatment entirely, feeling he is being justly punished. A person involved in faith healing may be convinced that her faith simply wasn't strong enough. She didn't pray long enough. She didn't trust enough in God.

Barbara Sigmund realistically said that the odds were better than even that she would die, and that it simply wouldn't help to do the rah-rah-sis-boom-bah routine and assure her that she could beat the odds if she only learned to love herself enough. She insisted that if she died she did not want to feel like a failure.

The influence of the mind is indeed great. If it could be mobilized appropriately, it might indeed be able to help a patient, at least psychologically. But denying the problem can be equally detrimental.

The Destructive Force of Denial

For those who are caught up in a "think yourself well" philosophy, the power of denial is great. Deniers minimize their symptoms and pain. A denying heart patient may feel pain but insist it's only heartburn or a sore muscle. "I must have worked out too hard," he says, and so disregards the symptom.

Denial alleviates the patient's mind, but his condition remains untreated. It has been estimated that the failure to recognize warning symptoms contributes to undue delay in seeking medical care in as many as 30 to 40 percent of heart attack patients. Yet denial is the only way some people can live with the guilt forced upon them by those who insist they could heal themselves with a positive mental attitude.

The Emotional Damage to Relatives

The emotional harm caused by alternative care isn't limited to patients. It also effects family and friends. Consider Mary Jane.

When she was forty, Mary Jane's doctors gave her a death sentence: She had terminal cancer. Although she had only months to live, she so distrusted the medical profession that she refused to try to prolong her life with chemotherapy. Instead, she sent her two young children to live with relatives across the country, left her husband at home, and went to a highly controversial—and very expensive—clinic in Mexico.

The clinic in Mexico cost Mary Jane $10,000 a week. Her treatment was to last four weeks. When she arrived back home, her husband says he hardly recognized her. "She was so thin and yellow. I could hardly believe she was my wife."

It cost Mary Jane $40,000 to spend the last month of her life in misery. "Sure, I'm resentful," her husband says today, five years after Mary Jane's death. "She chose to spend her last month down there instead of with her family. The doctors told us right out they couldn't cure her, but they may have been able to prolong her life. They certainly could have increased the quality of her last days."

4. Wasted Money

Mary Jane wasn't unique in the money she spent on alternative medicine. Neither was Gilda Radner. The American public spends approximately *4 billion dollars a year* on unproven cancer cures.

Is an unproven drug worth the cost? Can a clinic in Mexico accomplish what cannot be done in our country?

Neither patients nor their physicians can know everything about everything. I can't know about all the latest advances in chemotherapy. I don't know all the most recent changes in psychotherapy. I can't know how to perform all kinds of surgery. But what I can do is keep up on the scientific literature. I can educate my patients. And I can work with them to guide them to specialists who do know the latest information.

Working as a guide, educator, and counselor is an area in which alternative practitioners pride themselves. The problem is, they have abdicated any position of authority they may have had to their patients' intuition. This is often what they rely upon to decide which therapies will work. If the patient decides on iridology (diagnosis from an examination of the irises of the eyes), fine. If he or she chooses the occultic practice of contacting spirit guides, fine. It's up to the patient.

Because they don't speak from a position of authority, alternative practitioners do their patients a disservice. Patients don't know who to believe or who to trust. When a person picks up a compendium such as the *Encyclopedia of Alternative Health Care,* he generally thumbs through, looking for whatever makes sense to him. It was macrobiotics that jumped out at Gilda Radner. Never mind that there was no basis for it in scientific fact; it made sense to her, so it was a valid choice.

Too many people believe that the higher the price, the more valuable the product. This is a terribly unreliable gauge of the value of health practices.

5. Physical Threats

Physical threats, such as a nutritional deficiency, are particularly hazardous for cancer patients like Gilda Radner who try macrobiotics. Radner didn't embrace a macrobiotic diet right away, only once the cancer seemed to be gaining ground.

Gilda's physician prescribed a drug for her, which gave her a 10 to 15 percent chance that it would retard her cancer. She took the chance. But it wasn't enough.

Gilda then wanted to go to Mexico and take the Laetrile treatment too. But, she said, when her husband found out, "He flipped out. He had just had it. He said, 'No! Absolutely not!'"

Gilda thought, *He's abandoning me*. She fluctuated. She decided she would go to Mexico, with or without his support. All the while, she was growing more and more skeptical of medical treatments. Terrified, she'd wake up in the night screaming, "I'm going to die! I'm going to die!"

Gilda didn't go to Mexico. She continued with the chemotherapy, but people kept talking and she kept listening. A man in Connecticut told her about macrobiotic diets. These diets consist of large (macro) amounts of whole grains, especially brown rice, which are eaten in a meditative state. Macrobiotics is much more than just a restrictive diet. It becomes a way of life, dominating one's thoughts and actions. Of the group of cancer patients Gilda invited to her house for sharing and support, four were on macrobiotics.

Gee, food has always been a problem with me, Gilda thought. *Maybe food is the answer to getting well.*

Gilda became obsessed with macrobiotic books. She even had a gas stove installed so she could cook macrobiotically. She bought whole grains, seaweed, tofu, everything on the list. She even saw a macrobiotic counselor.

"You have a chance to recover," the macrobiotic counselor told Gilda.

This was the best news she ever heard.

Gilda's diet was specific: miso soup, rice cream five or six times a day, certain root vegetables three days on, three days off. She went "completely nutty" over macrobiotics. Only cotton clothes, the program said, so she threw away all clothing made of other fibers. No jewelry, it said. She threw away her jewelry. She also threw away her nail polish and changed all her cosmetics to "natural" products, as advised by the macrobiotic program. She walked on stones in the driveway to help her intestines. She quit talking on the phone and answering her mail because it was draining her energy. She focused only on herself. No one was allowed to come near her while she was eating: It was a meditative activity. She began to lose about a pound a day, going from 116 pounds down to 93.

Gilda continued to see her oncologist, but more and more

she was becoming disillusioned with him. He was impersonal, she said, and he seldom treated her as an individual. She felt that he looked at her and saw her dying. She had her husband call him and tell him she would not be coming back. Instead, she would stay with what she believed in: macrobiotics.

Gilda became involved with a psychologist who was interested in psychic healing. She attended two of his healing sessions. *What can it hurt?* she figured.

Meanwhile, she continued to insist she was getting better. She felt she was in outerspace—pure, blessed by God, sure that the cancer was disappearing from her body. But all the time the cancer was growing.

By the time Gilda finally agreed to see a new doctor, Dr. Greenspan, she was weak from the macrobiotic diet. Greenspan encouraged her to eat more. In a positive way, he assured her that things could be done to help the way she felt.

It was then that "a little door" opened for Gilda. She had shut herself off from the real world, in a little room of anger and fear and magical thinking. Now, she suddenly felt that there was a chance she could live and feel good without being on macrobiotics.

Under the doctor's care, Gilda began to feel better. Her weight went back up to 114 pounds, and her blood tests looked better.

Like many people, Gilda had wanted answers and results. Even though the rigid macrobiotic diet alienated her from her family and friends and almost killed her, Gilda had felt good about "taking action against the disease." She finally went full circle in her quest for a cure, from conventional medicine to the alternative methods, which almost killed her, and back to a caring and scientific physician. In most cases—even the most serious—something can be done to help. Just be sure your efforts do not lead to the physical harm and spiritual deception so common among the alternative medical practices.

Two years after being diagnosed, on October 3, 1988, Gilda had her final surgery. She died six months later. Did modern medicine ultimately fail her? The answer is no, unless you believe we should all live forever.

What about Laetrile?

Laetrile is another example of the potential physical harm that can come from so-called benign alternative treatments.

An extract from apricot pits, Laetrile has been one of the most widely investigated and tested cancer remedies of all time. In every test it has been found to be absolutely worthless. Even so, in its heyday 50,000 to 75,000 Americans took the drug. Reports of its miraculous cures were constantly circulated by individuals, media reports, talk shows, Tijuana cancer clinics, and alternative health advocates such as the National Health Federation (NHF)—all screaming for patients' right of "freedom of choice."

The testimonials were vivid and inspiring, and they packed tremendous dramatic impact. What they lacked was scientific validity.

NHF donated $5,000 toward the legal expenses of little Chad Green, a three-year-old with leukemia, and an NHF governor served as a lawyer for his parents. Chad attracted nationwide attention when his family moved to Mexico to avoid a Massachusetts court order to stop his Laetrile therapy and give him proper treatment.

The October 1979 issue of *Public Scrutiny* described how well the little boy was doing and how his father was studying for a career as a "nutrition consultant." A few days after the newspaper was distributed, the boy died. An autopsy revealed recurrent leukemia. There was also cyanide in his liver and spleen.

Dr. William Nolen, surgeon and author of such books as *Making of a Surgeon* and *Healing: A Doctor in Search of a Miracle,* tells of a thirty-five-year-old mother of three he diagnosed with early, treatable cancer of the uterus. He recommended surgery or radiation, but instead, she chose to go to

Mexico and spend $3,000 on Laetrile treatment. When she returned to him six months later, the cancer had spread to her pelvis, bladder, and rectum. She died one month later.

A California woman found a lump in her breast. Although she had no idea whether it was malignant or benign, she refused surgery to remove it. Instead, she went to a dispenser of Laetrile in Northern California, a man whose medical license was later rescinded, and paid him $3,500 for injections and tablets. She then returned to Southern California and continued to treat herself. After two episodes of cyanide poisoning, the woman was found to have inoperable breast cancer.

Are Vaccinations and Immunizations Harmful?

Another big physical problem posed by the alternative health movement is their opposition to mandatory vaccinations and immunizations. A variety of alternative practitioners, including some M.D.s, homeopaths, and naturopaths, are convincing parents that the general practice of vaccination may have long-term damaging effects on the immune system.

Richard Moskowitz, M.D., homeopath, and the former president of the National Center for Homeopathy, says, "All vaccinations may be injurious to the functioning and integrity of the immune system." Vaccinations involve injecting a minute amount of the disease-causing agent into the body—and homeopaths believe the more diluted a medicine, the more powerful it becomes.

But on what data is such a conclusion based? Is it derived from information or intuition? With advice like this, it's no wonder many patients today are confused about the need for vaccinations. In fact, Dr. Philip Inkao, a physician in New York who practices what he calls "anthroposophic" medicine, opposes vaccination on the ground that the struggle with infectious disease during childhood is beneficial to the child's personal and spiritual development.[9]

We invite Dr. Inkao to express his opinions to the thousands of children who have needlessly and permanently been crippled by polio. Childhood diseases are still a significant public health problem which require prevention.

Unfortunately, many well-meaning parents are bypassing childhood vaccinations by claiming exemptions on religious grounds, something that is permitted in all states except West Virginia and Mississippi. The problems posed by these unprotected children are great indeed.

Other Unorthodox "Treatments"

A recent article in the *American Medical News* (September 27, 1990) reported that a physician lost his license in New York after attempting to cure a woman's breast cancer with soft boiled eggs. He led three patients to believe he could cure their cancers and talked them out of seeking other care. A woman in her sixties sought him out after hearing on a radio program that he treated breast cancer without surgery. For about three years, in addition to the eggs, he treated her with vinegar, baking soda, and coffee. Although the doctor advised her against it, the woman eventually went to a hospital emergency room where her condition was diagnosed as breast cancer which had spread to her spine. If she had survived for three years, chances are that her original breast cancer was operable and curable. Her quack doctor robbed her of this chance for life.

A study on the use of unorthodox medical treatments in cancer patients found that one-third of those choosing unorthodox therapy alone had highly treatable types of cancer such as breast cancer. These were not last stage, terminal patients. Many of them could have survived their cancer.

6. Toxic Effects

The direct toxic effects of therapies include contaminated products, vitamin overdoses, and colonic cleansing enemas. While most alternative therapies don't kill, any time a substance is ingested, whether it is a natural preparation or not, there is the possibility of side effects. It's interesting, then, that so many therapists claim their concoctions are absolutely free of side effects.

The *American Journal of Public Health,* 1990, reports six deaths directly related to bacteria contaminated dried ground rattlesnake. Users were led to believe the capsules could treat AIDS, arthritis, cancer, infections and blood disorders.

Herbal products are especially prone to contamination by bacteria and fungi, as Laetrile was. Also, because these products are not carefully governed by the Federal Drug Administration, there is always the possibility of mislabeling.

The only time there is no possibility of side effects from a medication is when there is absolutely nothing in it, as is the case in many homeopathic mixtures so diluted nothing remains but water. And to risk contamination and toxic effects from unproven, untested potions is foolish indeed. The next time someone attempts to convince you that any "all-natural" food, nutrient, or potion must be inherently good for you because it is untainted by mankind, remind them that several natural substances, like hemlock, also fall into this category.

Both special diet regimens, like the one Gilda Radner adopted, and metabolic therapies put people at risk of suffering toxic effects. It is reported that fully 20 percent of all cancer patients take megadoses of vitamins. Not only is this useless; excessive vitamins can actually be poisonous and add further irritation to an already stressed body.

Laetrile is also a good example of the potential toxic effects of unregulated substances. Vials of injectable Laetrile were found to be contaminated with bacteria and fungi. Even more frightening, evidence began to surface that Laetrile smuggled in from Mexico contained potentially deadly levels of cyanide. A toxicologist from the Federal Drug Administration reported that many cancer patients who had taken long-term high doses of Laetrile actually died of slow cyanide poisoning!

7. Diverted Resources

Despite what some may think, our country has limited resources with which to fight disease and provide preventive health care. Even though ours is a rich country which spends billions of dollars each year—11 percent of our gross national product—on health care, there's never enough money. If we divert funds into questionable areas, we will have that much less for legitimate research and therapy.

Again, Laetrile is a good example of what happens. Although it had already been proven on numerous occasions to be ineffective in the treatment of cancer, the lobbying efforts of certain individuals gained the ear of congressmen who were able to get hundreds of thousands of additional research dollars—spent, as it turned out, on proving Laetrile was indeed ineffective.

Because AIDS is such an emotionally and politically charged issue, AIDS research is ripe for particular abuse. Dr. John Renner, a Kansas city family physician and consumer advocate, has for the past seven years been actively involved in exposing the dangers of quackery and health scams. He is particularly concerned with the rampant AIDS quackery. It has become a more fertile ground even than cancer. Although AIDS doesn't strike as many people, it has a more definitive and hopeless outlook.

A new and truly disturbing wrinkle is insurance companies' agreement to pay for what can at best be called questionable therapies. Eventually, even Mary Jane's bill from the Mexican clinic was paid in full by her insurance company. What this means is that we—all of us—are supporting alternative practitioners and their practices through our insurance premiums. We don't know about you, but we strongly resent contributing our hard earned money to such quackery.

8. Loss of Reality

In many alternative medical practices, reality has assumed an entirely new meaning. Now reality is relative. It is whatever a person perceives it to be. "Don't intervene," families are told when they question a particular therapy. "If you don't support her, the therapy won't work." As a family practice resident in Charleston, South Carolina, I was called to the emergency room to see a patient who was bleeding from her breast. She was surrounded by her obviously loving and concerned family—her husband, who was a distinguished looking, high ranking navy officer, and a high-school-aged son and daughter. The woman was pale, and in a great deal of pain. When I pulled the towel back from her chest, I was horrified to see an enormous, bleeding mass, exuding from her left breast. The bleeding was so great that it couldn't be controlled by the towels. Her breast itself was swollen to the size of a large cantaloupe. Never had I seen such an advanced case of cancer.

In absolute shock and amazement, I asked the patient, "Why did you wait so long to get help?" When she didn't answer, I asked her distraught family, "Why didn't you make her come sooner?"

They told me they had agreed to support her decision to rely upon prayer for healing. She believed if it was God's will for her to get well, she would. They simply prayed she would "do the right thing." Family support didn't heal this woman. Neither did her strong belief in God. Demanding healing from God on your own arbitrary terms makes you bedfellows with New Agers who also demand to be in charge with "create your own reality" thinking. We believe God can work through competent physicians and we should take advantage of this provision.

Certainly, any of us confronted with confusing and emotionally disturbing information can blunder into a foolish course of action. In such a case, Richard Ofshe, a University of California at Berkeley professor who won a Pulitzer prize for his research on the Synanon cult, suggests "reality testing." He recommends asking the following questions:

1. What is the theory behind the program or technique?
2. How do the procedures relate to the theory?
3. Are there objective criteria for evaluation?

Many people approach alternative health care with the idea that a retreat into a fantasy world is preferable to painful reality. Gilda Radner withdrew from everything, including her friends. She wouldn't even eat with her husband because of the macrobiotic suggestion that it was energy draining to eat with another person. Mary Jane left her husband and two young children and spent $40,000 they couldn't afford in her futile search for a cure. Patients go through torment seeking new reality in alternative treatments.

Failure to diagnose. Failure to treat. Physical threats. Toxic effects. Emotional harm. Wasted money. Diverted resources. Loss of reality. Can alternative health practices really hurt? Absolutely! They can hurt, and they can kill.

The final danger of alternative health care is the spiritual harm. We will discuss that in the next chapter.

Chapter Three

JUST SPIT OUT THE BAD

Don't Worry about
Spiritual Harm?

When I read Dr. Bernie Siegel's book *Love, Medicine and Miracles* and realized the spiritual influences within his philosophy, I thought it would be good to discuss the book with our local Christian physicians group at our monthly meeting. At the beginning of the meeting I asked, "How many of you have heard of Bernie Siegel?"

Many raised their hands. A good number indicated they had read his book. What surprised me was how many felt positive about it.

"He talks a lot about love," they said. "He speaks about the power of positive thinking, about encouraging your patients, about how to deal more effectively with bad circumstances." They liked all of that. The general consensus was that Siegel was doing okay.

Page by page, I went through the book with them, showing how, in his own words, Siegel pushed the idea of altered states of consciousness. When discussing meditation, he writes, "I know of no other single activity that by itself can produce such a great improvement in the quality of life"[1]

I pointed out the way in which patients could easily become

tools for shamans and yogis. (He tells of an African delegate to the United Nations who had been told by a New York doctor that he had cancer and would die within a year. According to the delegate, soon after he returned home to Africa, the local witch doctor began therapy. From a large cauldron he dipped a small cup of liquid and said, "This cup represents the part of your brain you are using. The cauldron the rest. I will teach you to use the rest." Today, Dr. Siegel says, the man is alive and well.[2])

I warned about the author's push for the acquisition of power animals and spirit guides. (He contends his own personal spirit guide is "George, a bearded, long-haired young man wearing an immaculate flowing white gown and skullcap."[3])

I warned about the book's favorable references to mediums and familiar spirits. (One night, while giving a lecture, Siegel says he began to realize that he was actually giving two talks—one, from the prepared outline before him, and the other, something unexpected coming unbidden from him. The second was much better, so he finally gave in and let the unprepared talk take over. After the lecture, a woman came up to him and said, " 'I'm a medium, and while you were reading Lois Becker's letter, superimposed over you and staring at the audience was this figure. I drew him for you.' And she showed me a picture of my guide George."[4] It would seem that Dr. Siegel is completely unable to recognize the occultic nature of spirit guides.)

I talked about Siegel's belief in reincarnation, his association with occultists and psychics, and his communication with the dead and encouragement of the same in his patients. (He reports that a woman told him of a dream "in which Death came and told her that her husband was going to die tomorrow. She argued with Death and said, 'No. Everybody gets two weeks' notice.' Two weeks to the day later her husband died."[5])

How did these Christian doctors feel about Siegel now? Some of them were surprised. Yet, interestingly enough, some were still of the opinion that the good in Siegel's message outweighed the bad.

Unfortunately, that's not the first time I've heard this Watergate-type of reasoning. An interfaith witness director for the Home Mission Board of the Southern Baptist Convention expressed the same opinion. A supposed expert on the New Age movement, he was teaching at a church in North Carolina that was riddled with dissension over New Age health practices, especially iridology and applied kinesiology. Here's what he had to say about Dr. Bernie Siegel: "It's a lot like eating fish with bones. Just spit out the bones."

"Just spit out the bad." "The good in his message outweighed the bad."

Don't believe it. It's not nearly as easy to separate the good from the bad as some would have us believe. And, believe me, the good in no way outweighs the bad. The fact is, the good is so contaminated with the bad that it cannot possibly be of any use to anyone except for its owner to deceive.

This same gentleman, in an effort to appear even-handed, actually suggested that totally invalid and deceptive practices such as iridology, applied kinesiology and reflexology might actually be acceptable if presented in a "Christian frame of reference." I suppose this means we should consider the possibility that the popular, occult work *A Course in Miracles* is really acceptable because the spirit who channeled this three-volume work claimed to be Jesus.

Whether they realize it or not, those who become involved in the alternative health movement are getting a religious message. In many cases, they are being indoctrinated directly into the world of the occult. Much within alternative health care, and many of those who practice and teach it, are cunningly deceptive. Perhaps that deception is the greatest danger of all.

So here we are, back at deception. The deception of alternative health care is twofold. It entails

1. the belief that a patient can rely totally on alternative health care and without giving it a second thought; and
2. the spiritual deception perpetrated by Eastern mysticism and occultism.

For many people who are simply seeking better health, New

Age medicine becomes their entry into the religious aspects of the New Age movement. Kristin Olsen, in her recent book on alternative health care, clearly states the holistic health movement's religious bent: "Many professional health care providers integrate Chinese or Indian medicine-based philosophy or Buddhist spiritual principles into a Western health approach."[6]

Alternative health care is nothing but a commonsense, unified system of health care, you thought? Think again. Spiritual harm comes from the trickery which entices a person to become involved in Eastern mysticism and occultic practices without realizing it.

Alternative medicine is a call for a completely new way of caring for the sick. It's a call for a radically new way of looking at our world.

Alternative medicine—which also goes by the name of New Age medicine—is often the entree for people who are searching for this new world view. Marilyn Ferguson, author of *The Aquarian Conspiracy,* wrote that "the impending transformation of medicine is a window to the transformation of all our institutions." It is precisely this fact that makes alternative medicine so important—and so dangerous.

WHAT IS 'THE NEW AGE'?

When it comes to New Age, strict definitions don't mean much. The New Age movement is an umbrella term which covers a multitude of seemingly disparate groups, quite literally from A (aromatherapy) to Z (Zen Buddhism). Rather than being a cohesive movement, it is exceedingly diverse in its makeup and its ideology. The factors that unite the New Age factions are their shared beliefs rather than a shared organization.

New Age expert Bob Larson, in his book *Straight Answers on the New Age,* defines the New Age movement as "a networking of individuals and organizations dedicated to a mystical interpretation of reality and the pursuance of occult practices to enhance spirituality."[7]

New Age visionaries see the world and all of humanity preparing to make a cosmic leap into a future millennial world of
peace and prosperity. They see the attainment of a higher consciousness and inner healing as essential stepping stones to the
Nirvana of the New Age. Through spiritual and holistic health
practices, a "paradigm shift"—a new definition of reality—will
supposedly occur. The result will be a change in all of society's
institutions.

Because most alternative care practitioners are willing to accept almost any form of treatment—regardless of whether or
not it is scientifically valid—the variations of the holistic theme
are endless. Nevertheless, certain themes come up again and
again.

SPIRITUAL THEMES IN ALTERNATIVE
HEALTH CARE

Let's look at how alternative health care reflects the "spirituality" of New Age thinking.

New Age Belief 1: All Is One

This is not all for one and one for all, as in the Three Muske-
teers. No, this New Age philosophy states literally, *all is one*.
Everything and everyone is interrelated and interdependent. In
the end, there really is no difference between you and me.
There is no difference between people and animals, between
humans and rocks, between the Creator and the creation. Sure,
we think there are differences, but they are merely perceived.
This concept, known as monism, is central to many Eastern
religions. Now it pervades the concept of disease in the alternative health movement.

Holism

If one central principle permeates the alternative health care
movement, it is holism—the unity of body, mind, and spirit. On
the surface, this concept sounds like plain old common sense.

But alternative health care promoters now present this thought either as an entirely new revelation, or as a return to what they term "intuitive intelligence."

As Christian health professionals, the thought of helping a person in all three of these important areas greatly appeals to us. But the New Age health movement sees this unity quite differently than we do. Body, mind, and spirit are not merely recognized as interrelated parts of a person but in terms of the concept "All is one." Thus, personal godhood is only a moment's meditation away.

In considering the implications of the holistic concept of health care, Christian professionals are reminded of Jesus' own words: "I have come that they may have life, and that they may have it more abundantly" (John 10:10). But for New Agers, the potential for the abundant life within you is the same as the divine life force.

The New Age god is impersonal energy or whatever your intuition tells you God is. This Eastern concept of God is woven throughout alternative medicine. Bernie Siegel says God is "an intelligent, loving energy or light—in each person's life."[8] Siegel, the medical theologian, goes on to tell us that illness is a sin. "I suggest that patients think of illness not as God's will but as our deviation from God's will."[9]

Physicians who have long recognized the physical and emotional needs of mankind are increasingly sensing the spiritual side of themselves and their patients. This we applaud. But just as strongly we argue against the unbiblical presentation of God as an impersonal energy force or a product of our "collective unconscious."

All of the "force" or "energy" medical practices—such as acupuncture, reflexology, and therapeutic touch—are based on the belief that there is a universal life force running through all people which connects them to all other forms in the universe, and ultimately to the universe itself. If you balance your yin and yang, if you adjust your bio-force, if you heal your chi, then and only then can true healing occur.

Energy

To many holistic healers, poor health is nothing more than an energy crisis. Belief in the flow of "universal energy" through each individual, each plant, and each animal, through the earth and the cosmos, ultimately connecting each living person with the entire universe, is central to many of the current New Age healing practices. This energy attains God-like proportions when attributes such as omnipresence and "basis for all life" are given to it.

Many holistic practices base their entire ability to diagnose and treat disease on the practitioner's ability to detect blockages of this unseen, unproven, unmeasurable force. These practitioners are convinced that only by the release of this blocked energy can true health be achieved. How can this energy be manipulated? The methods are limited only by the imaginations of the healers and their desperate patients.

"Reiki" is an example of this type of therapy. By laying on of hands, Reiki therapists harmonize themselves and people on whom they work with Universal Life Energy. "This great Cosmos Energy is present everywhere. It is limitless. It makes life possible. It can revitalize and restore inner peace. . . . Therapists recharge the body, building up energy wherever tension or disease has set. Diseased organs soak up the life force that flows through the therapist's hands, penetrating deep into organs that need it. Energy continues to build until sufficient enough to break through blocks."[10]

For Reiki, we could substitute any number of holistic health practices based on the manipulation of universal energy or force: therapeutic touch, reflexology, acupuncture, yoga, applied kinesiology, jin shin do, crystal therapy—they all have the same basic philosophy. Although new terms, such as bio-plasma or "the Force" as depicted in George Lucas' Star Wars trilogy, are constantly being introduced, all draw heavily from ancient concepts of Eastern mysticism.

Seeking to legitimize and validate their belief in this energy flowing through the universe, the disciples of energy medicine have found willing partners in the field of modern physics. Fritjof Capra, author of *The Tao of Physics,* and Deepak Chopra, who wrote *Quantum Healing* are typical of those attempting to marry Eastern mysticism with modern quantum mechanics. By the millions, Westerners are being advised that the way to health and happiness is through practices which are in reality no more than ancient Eastern religious concepts. The difference is that they are disguised in pseudo-scientific terms and settings.

Accepting the various theories and methods for manipulating "universal energy" is but a short step from the Hindu teachings espoused in the cult following of Transcendental Meditation. Maharishi Mahesh Yogi speaks in his book *Science of Being and Art of Living* of the "enlightened" understanding of God (energy) in you and you as energy (God). Unfortunately, when this theory is put to the ultimate test, it falls woefully short. A report in the TM-Ex *News* (Fall, 1990) tells of a student at Maharishi International University in Fairfield, Iowa, who was killed by a speeding train. He was trying to stop it with Transcendental Meditation.

New Age Belief 2: All Is God

Once you have accepted the idea that all is one, you're ready to embrace pantheism—that is, *everything is god*. It's the next logical assumption. All of life—even all of non-life—has a spark of divinity within. Alternative practitioners frequently talk about the "innate intelligence" within us all. If we can only tap into this intelligence, we can heal ourselves. Often described as "the inner physician," this mystical healing force is hailed as the ultimate power behind all physical healing.

Mind Over Disease

"Ultimately, you yourself are responsible for your own health." This is the distinctive message of alternative medicine. The Hindus believe in the concept of maya, that a person creates his own reality. Carried to the extreme, personal responsibility for illness is the medical version of maya. Dr. Gerald Epstein states in his book *Healing Visualizations— Creating Healing Through Imagery,* that illness is nothing more than a state of forgetting how to be whole. By simply remembering, one can be well again. What comforting news this must be to the mother of a child with a congenital birth defect!

Alternative health care is packed with examples of this mind over disease approach. Christian Science healing—actually neither Christian nor scientific—is a classic example of the think-yourself-well mentality. Christian Scientists simply deny that illness exists—so it doesn't. Right?

Not according to some who have tried it. In April of 1986, two-and-a-half year old Robyn Twitchell died in terrible pain five days after the onset of a bowel obstruction. In July of 1990, at his parents' trial in Boston, Christian Science attorneys claimed the Twitchells were not on trial. Their religion was. David Twitchell agreed. "This has been a prosecution against our faith," he proclaimed. Yet in a more poignant moment he sadly voiced his misgivings: "If medicine could have saved him I wish I had turned to it." Doctors say the boy's condition could have been cured. The jury agreed and convicted the parents of manslaughter.[11]

The desire for personal responsibility, and the demand that each person (or the child's parents) determine his own medical course, comes with a terrifyingly high price tag—the guilty realization that not getting well is also a personal responsibility. People with incurable diseases flock to medical messiahs of eternal optimism and hope. If they can just take enough vitamins, if they can only meditate a little more deeply, if they can achieve greater powers of visualization—then health and vitality can again be theirs. How deep must be their despair, and how great their personal guilt, when their bodies don't respond.

Without a doubt, the omnipotent God is everywhere. But everything, the Bible tells us, is certainly not God. To insist that everything is God is the beginning of idolatry. Remember God's first commandment to the Israelites? "You shall have no other gods before Me" (Ex. 20:3). "No other gods" includes you yourself.

God demands no less from us today.

New Age Belief 3: You Are God

If all is one, and if all is God, then the next logical progression is that *we are all gods*. All people are one with the entire universe, and all are one with God. God is then reduced to an impersonal force or consciousness.

Reducing God from Almighty Creator to a mere part of the great universe is a radical departure from the Christian concept of a personal God, the loving, caring Creator of all things. The Bible says: "For by Him all things were created that are in heaven and that are on earth, visible and invisible. . . . All things were created through Him and for Him" (Col. 1:16).

To New Agers, that we are all God is a given. The only problem, say New Age authors and teachers, is that we are ignorant of our own divinity. They refer to all of us as "Gods in disguise." Transcendental Meditation (TM) is an example of this concept transferred to the alternative health care arena. The untapped potential of self-realization is the goal of devotees of TM. Believing in their true divinity, meditators seek higher consciousness and inner healing. Once you attain this consciousness, they claim, you will finally recognize that you yourself are a god.

The goal of the New Age Movement is that each of us come to the place where we discover our own divinity. We accomplish this by experiencing a change in consciousness. The human race suffers from a collective form of metaphysical amnesia, New Agers teach. We have forgotten that our true identity is divine. That's why we need to undergo a change of consciousness before we can achieve our true human potential (hence the name "The Human Potential Movement"). Christian Scientists and other alternative healing cults teach that recognition of inner divinity negates the reality of physical illness.

New Age Belief 4: Reincarnation

Most New Agers believe in some form of reincarnation. In its classic form, the cycles of birth, death, and reincarnation are necessary to work off our "bad karma" and finally allow us to reach perfection. The doctrine of karma says that one's present condition was determined by one's actions in a past life.

The Western version of reincarnation held by many New Agers places much less emphasis on bad karma. Instead it teaches an upward spiral toward perfection through reincarnation. This is the view espoused by such people as Shirley MacLaine, Sylvester Stallone, George Patton, and Henry Ford—and a good many others whose names are not so well known. New Age medicine points to those who have had near-death experiences (NDE) as proof of reincarnation—a position that replaces the Christian belief in eternal life with God after death.

Near Death Experiences

For many in our society, death is the greatest of mysteries. It awaits us all. Many are not only curious, but are desperate to learn more about it.

Dr. Elisabeth Kübler-Ross, who has contributed much to our understanding of the dying process, is also an avowed believer in reincarnation. She says that "To work with dying patients has helped me to find my own religious identity, to know that there is life after death and to know that we will be reborn again one day in order to complete the tasks we have not been able or willing to complete in this lifetime."[12]

Dr. Kübler-Ross works closely with Raymond Moody, M.D., Ph.D., psychiatrist and author of the best-selling book *Life After Life*. (Dr. Moody is the originator of the term "near death experience" (NDE), and founder of the International Association of Near Death Studies.) Both Kübler-Ross and Moody are deeply involved in researching out-of-body and near death experiences documented from a variety of people who have been pronounced clinically dead but were later revived. Drawing from 150 interviews, Dr. Moody summarized them in a composite after death experience:

A man is dying and, as he reaches the point of greatest physical distress, he hears himself pronounced dead by his doctor. He begins to hear an uncomfortable noise, a loud ringing or buzzing, and at the same time feels himself moving very rapidly through a long dark tunnel. After this, he suddenly finds himself outside of his own physical body, but still in the immediate physical environment, and sees his own body from a distance as though he is a spectator. He watches the resuscitation attempt from this unusual vantage point and is in a state of emotional upheaval. After a while, he collects himself and becomes more accustomed to his odd condition. He notices that he still has a body; but one of a very different nature and with very different powers from the physical body he has left behind. Soon other things begin to happen. Others come to meet and to help him. He glimpses the spirits of relatives and friends who have already died, and a loving, warm spirit of a kind he has never encountered before—a being of light—appears before him. This being asks him a question, nonverbally, to make him evaluate his life and helps him along by showing him a panoramic, instantaneous playback of the major events of his life. At some point he finds himself approaching some sort of barrier or border, apparently representing the limit between earthly life and the next life. Yet he finds that he must go back to the earth, that the time for his death is not yet come. At this point he resists, for by now he is taken up with his experiences in the after life and does not want to return. He is overwhelmed by intense feelings of joy, love, and peace. Despite this attitude, though, he somehow reunites with his physical body and lives.[13]

According to a book by Barbara Harris, a research assistant at the University of Connecticut Health Center in Farmington, and author of the book *Full Circle, The Near Death Experience and Beyond,* fully eight million Americans say they have had a near death experience. One of the compelling aspects of this phenomenon is the consistency of the accounts—the out-of-body experience, the peace, the tunnel, the light, the life review, the deceased relatives or spirits who come to the individual. Dr. Moody has himself interviewed over 1,000 people who have had NDEs, and has identified nine characteristic traits, which he says typify them.

1. A sense of being dead.
2. Peace and painlessness.
3. An out-of-body experience.
4. A tunnel experience.
5. People of light.
6. A being of light.
7. A life review.
8. A reluctance to return.
9. Personality transformation.

That changes take place in individuals who have had an NDE is obvious in the stories of many people who have gone through this. One, Steve Price, a Vietnam veteran, says that after an NDE he became curious about a variety of things, including quantum mechanics and Buddhism, and a wide range of paranormal phenomena including reincarnation, UFOs, and auras. Price says he also developed the ability to heal simply by placing his hands on a painful area. He claims to have healed his wife's tension headaches and a cat's sore ear.[14]

The similarities between the near death experiences and the "shamanic journey" are more than coincidental. Michael Harner, a shaman (spiritual guide) and author of *The Way of the Shaman,* states that the classic description of the shamanic journey involves the path to the underworld via a tunnel, much like the tunnel experienced in near death experiences. He says this journey is achieved through an altered state of consciousness. This is something that also happens for those in a near death experience. A catastrophe has happened, something like being struck by lightning, nearly drowning, or experiencing a cardiac arrest.

One rather frightening aspect of the shamanic journey is a statement by Shaman Harner who says that on one occasion when he had undergone a journey, he had the distinct impression that something had come back with him. It was right behind him, he says. "It was beneficial or benevolent. It was not bad." Now, just what this was, or how he determined whether it was bad or good, is up for debate.

No Death, No Judgment

Interestingly, those doing research into near death experiences almost always report benign trips and good experiences. Very seldom does anyone report negative experiences.

One writer who has delved into negative near death experiences is Dr. Maurice Rawlings, a specialist in internal medicine and cardiovascular disease who wrote *Beyond Death's Door*. Dr. Rawlings writes that "many people have wondered why recently reported experiences (of NDEs) all seem to be good ones. They've asked why after death experiences do not also represent unpleasant or bad experiences."[15] He said he personally has had many opportunities to resuscitate people who have clinically died, and in interviews immediately afterward, patients reveal as many bad experiences as good ones.

For example, Dr. Rawlings reported that in 1977 he resuscitated a terrified patient who told him he was in hell. He begged the doctor to get him out of hell and not to let him die. "When I fully realized how genuinely and extremely frightened he was, I too became frightened," writes Rawlings. "Subsequent cases with terrifying experiences have burdened me with a sense of urgency to write this book, *Beyond Death's Door*."[16]

Dr. Rawlings doesn't doubt for a minute the authenticity of the near death experiences. The events are so minutely and accurately recounted by patients that they suggest a spiritual existence outside the body during this period of clinical death. He relates an experience which occurred while the patient was undergoing a cardiac stress test to figure out what was causing his chest pains. The forty-eight year old rural postman was on a treadmill and hooked up to an electrocardiogram. During the test, his heart stopped beating and he dropped dead right in the doctor's office.

Dr. Rawlings immediately began cardio-pulminary resuscitation. Eventually he had to implant a pacemaker into the patient's heart. Finally the patient's heartbeat began to return on its own. Yet whenever Dr. Rawlings reached for an instrument or otherwise interrupted the chest compressions, the man began to lose consciousness. As soon as his heart began to beat again, he screamed, "I am in hell!"

This happened time and time again. Finally the man cried out, "Don't you understand? Each time you quit I go back to hell! Don't let me go back to hell!" The terrified patient pleaded with the doctor to help him.

It was this episode that encouraged Rawlings to write his book. He says that while he feels certain there is life after death, not all of it is good.

A couple days after this patient was hospitalized, Dr. Rawlings asked him about being in hell. The man said, "What hell? I don't recall any hell." Dr. Rawlings told the patient what had happened, but the man could recall none of the unpleasant events.

Apparently the experiences were so frightening, so horrible and painful, the conscious mind could not cope with them, and so they were suppressed far into the subconscious. Interestingly enough, although Dr. Rawlings' cardiac patient didn't remember screaming for the doctor to keep him out of hell, he did recall meeting both his mother and stepmother during the death experiences. The experience was very pleasurable, the patient insisted. It occurred in a narrow valley with lush vegetation and brilliant illumination by a huge beam of white.

Patients, Rawlings found, tend to remember only the pleasant details. It occurred to him that Dr. Kübler-Ross, Dr. Moody, and others were interviewing patients several days or even several weeks after they had been resuscitated. He believes that if patients could be interviewed immediately following their NDE, researchers would find as many bad experiences as good ones.

Rawlings' research points to a more biblical view, which insists that death will be followed by judgment. In the Bible God states that "It is appointed for men to die once, but after this the judgment" (Heb. 9:27). Near death experiences have been used by those who would claim that there is no death, or no judgment after death.

In September of 1976, Kübler-Ross stepped further out of the world of science and into the realm of the occult when she announced to an audience that she had acquired her own personal spirit guide by the name of Salem. At one speaking engagement she said, "Last night I was visited by Salem, my spirit guide, and two of his companions, Anka and Willie. They were with us until three o'clock in the morning. We talked, laughed, and sang together. They spoke and touched me with the most incredible love and tenderness imaginable. This was the highlight of my life."[17]

One of the key messages delivered both by those who have suffered near death experiences and out-of-body experiences is "You will not die." Do you hear a familiar ring? Genesis 3:1–5 says:

Now the serpent was more cunning than any beast of the field which the Lord God had made. And he said to the woman, "Has God indeed said, 'You shall not eat of every tree of the garden'?" And the woman said to the serpent, "We may eat the fruit of the trees of the garden; but of the fruit of the tree which is in the midst of the garden, God has said, 'You shall not eat it, nor shall you touch it, lest you die.'" And the serpent said to the woman, "You will not surely die. For God knows that in the day you eat of it your eyes will be opened, and you will be like God, knowing good and evil."

Christians have always been comforted by the thought that after they die, they will be reunited with Jesus Christ. The apostle Paul said:

Therefore we are always confident, knowing that while we are at home in the body we are absent from the Lord. For we walk by faith, not by sight. We are confident, yes, well pleased rather to be absent from the body and to be present with the Lord. Therefore we make it our aim, whether present or absent, to be well pleasing to Him (2 Cor. 5:6–9).

We know there is life after death. So why should we be surprised at these accounts of NDEs? Yet we must be careful about the conclusions we draw. Many assume that the bright light is God or Jesus. Not necessarily, for 2 Corinthians 11:14–15 tells that "Satan himself transforms himself into an angel of light. Therefore it is no great thing if his ministers also transform themselves into ministers of righteousness, whose end will be according to their works."

WHAT'S DIFFERENT TODAY?

Many people mistakenly assume that this fascination with alternative medicine is a relatively recent thing. Certainly, today we are all more aware of what is happening around us. But is this so-called New Age medicine really new?

Well, the terms are new. So are the organizations. Take the American Holistic Medical Association for instance. Founded just over ten years ago, this organization represents physicians with a holistic bent. The AHMA is now headquartered in Raleigh, North Carolina, and holds regular meetings. It offers approved continuing medical education credited by the American Medical Association on such topics as Shamanism, Spiritual Attunements, and the Electromagnetic Man.

But it's just the terms that have changed. When the tenets of the New Age Movement are examined, we find that they aren't new at all. New Age medicine is nothing more than age-old occultism dressed up in new linguistic garb. In fact, many of its concepts can be found in basic form in the third chapter of Genesis. Notice these statements the serpent made to Eve in the Garden of Eden: "You will be like God" (pantheism) . . . "You shall not surely die" (reincarnation) . . . "Your eyes will be opened" (enlightened through altered consciousness).

New Age philosophy in general, and New Age medicine in particular, are not really new at all.

Chapter Four

WHOM DO YOU CALL?

From the day Loretta's colon cancer was diagnosed, she was shuttled from specialist to specialist to specialist. First she saw her oncologist, a doctor who deals with the cancer. Then a proctologist, a radiologist, a pathologist, a gastroenterologist, an internal medicine specialist, an anesthesiologist, and a surgeon.

"I feel fragmented," Loretta said. "No one really cares about me. To them I'm just another cancer patient, nothing but a statistic."

Roy also feels fragmented. For almost two years, he has been going through medical tests. He is learning the frustrating truth we doctors already know: medicine is not an exact science and all the answers are not known. Sometimes, despite our most sophisticated tests, a diagnosis remains elusive. Roy has endured pricking and prodding, x-rays and body scans, endless blood tests and time-consuming examinations. And still the best we can do is tell him, "It's not all in your mind. There really is something wrong. We just don't know what it is."

Both Loretta and Roy have looked into alternative medicine

practitioners. The attraction for Loretta? "He saw me as a real person. Not a disease, but a human being. And that's how he treated me." Sounds familiar, doesn't it.

And Roy? "The holistic doctor had a diagnosis for me and has suggested a treatment. He said he could help me."

Many patients have complaints similar to those expressed by Loretta and Roy:

"My doctor wouldn't listen to me."

"He was always in a hurry."

"She's so impersonal, I don't even feel like I have a doctor."

"I'm going to too many doctors. I want just one who can deal with the whole me."

As a family physician who is called upon to see a wide variety of patients and problems, I recognize the need for coordination of the medical effort. But at the same time I see the need for specialty care. Each has an important place in scientific medicine. Alternative medicine offers an even more bewildering array of practitioners, from homeopaths and naturopaths to herbalists and colonic hygienists.

Yet I realize that misgivings about the medical establishment are growing. More and more people resent the authoritative, paternalistic, overbearing attitude that has become the trademark of some physicians. Mother Teresa, 1979 Nobel Prize recipient, said, "The biggest disease today is not leprosy or tuberculosis, but rather the feeling of being unwanted, uncared for and deserted by everybody."

Medical doctors have to bear some responsibility for the increase in alternative medicine. Some patients are seeking cures outside traditional medicine because we have let them down.

THE PATIENT'S NEED TO UNDERSTAND

"She is more than just an acupuncturist," Roy says of his latest therapist. "She's a friend."

Alternative practitioners appear willing to sit and listen. They encourage their patients to talk about all areas of their lives, not just the cancer or the x-ray or the latest blood test. They don't rush their patients or act impatient when the patients ask questions and air complaints.

Certainly it takes much more time to explain terms and conditions and tests to patients than just to write out a prescription and say, "Take two of these three times a day." But patients want to understand their conditions. They are looking for answers.

"With all the high tech equipment available today, I can't believe any condition could go on for two years without being diagnosed," says Roy.

Somebody comes along with a diagnosis or a treatment, and the exasperated patient is sold. Whatever the mode of therapy, if a "professional" tells about it enthusiastically and convincingly, desperate patients reach out and willingly become involved.

"What I liked was that it was something I could do for myself," Loretta said of the macrobiotic diet she was following enthusiastically. "I've felt helpless too long."

Physicians traditionally have ignored the concept of allowing the patient to be involved. They say, "Don't worry. You don't really need to understand. Just trust me." Or as a friend of ours who is a doctor's daughter tells us, "Mom always said to me, 'I can't give you a medical degree in an hour. It's just too complicated for you to understand.'" But the patient wants to understand. Physicians say, "Here, take this pill," or, "We'll call in a surgeon." So the pill goes to work and the surgeon goes to work; but what about the patient? What can she do?

"I just hate feeling helpless!" Loretta insists.

THE MAZE OF M.D.s

Another common complaint is the overspecialization of medicine.

"Who do I go to?" Roy asks in confusion. "Every doctor finishes his examinations and his tests and says, 'Well, it's nothing in my area. Good-bye and good luck.' I've been to a psychologist, a neurologist, an internist, and now a second neurologist, and it's always the same. So who do I go to next?"

"I once tried to talk to my doctor about nutrition," Loretta says. "He tore a sheet off a pad with some basic nutritional information on it—things like the basic food groups—and gave it to me. I don't think he knew any more about nutrition than I did. I guess they don't teach that in medical school."

So what did Loretta do? She sought out a "nutritionist," someone recommended by a clerk in her local health food store.

"The nutritionist told me good nutrition is important," Loretta continued, "but she said I also needed supplements. She gave me a whole list of things to get at the health food store." Unfortunately Loretta knew nothing about this nutritionist's qualifications or the effects of the supplements she recommended.

Alternative health care practitioners are good at speaking with authority. When asked a question, they don't hesitate. "Oh, yes, I know this works," they say. How do they know? "Because a man I know tried it and . . ." Their claims are seldom backed up with scientific studies. For them the best proof is anecdotal. They prefer exciting testimonials to solid, but boring research.

When a suffering middle-aged woman hears that a fifty-year-old woman with symptoms "just like hers" got well because she took certain vitamins, or because she tried a specific therapy, the woman accepts the remedy as proven. "Oh, she came right in here and told me about her suffering," the practitioner adds. "You should see her today!"

Alternative practitioners love to quote testimonials. They like to tell how many people have used this particular therapy—always successfully, of course. When you hear these recitations, it's important to keep in mind that testimonials, like statistics, can be made to say almost anything. Who conducted the interview? How was it conducted? Who selected the patient? Was that person one of many cases, or was he a real exception?

So whom *do* you call? Medical doctor? Chiropractor? Psychic healer? How is a person to choose? The more complex the health problem, the more difficult the choice.

WHOM DO YOU CALL?

It's not hard to decide what to do about a runny nose. A box of tissues and an over-the-counter decongestant is likely to do as much good as anything. Or perhaps the placebo effects of a hot bowl of chicken soup or a big glass of orange juice will fill the bill. But what about a really difficult-to-diagnose problem? Or one that is potentially life threatening?

Many people have someone they consider "my doctor," and they naturally go to that physician for medical care and advice. Increasingly, however, Americans are also looking to other healers out in the wings. They may have a chiropractor, perhaps, or a vitamin supplement sales clerk at the local health food store who advises them about pseudo-nutrition. Some may have an acupuncturist or a massage therapist. Some may go to a naturopathic physician.

So how does a wise consumer go about selecting health care practitioners and methods? It may not be so hard to weed out the overtly strange and occultic ones, but those who speak in scientific terminology, those white-coated professionals espousing medical jargon—how do we know about them? And what of those who call themselves Christian healers: Christian psychic healers, faith healers, Christian channelers, Christian meditation therapists, Christian nutritionists?

Randall Baer is a former naturopathic doctor and internationally known New Age author and authority on crystals who has rejected the alternative medicine movement. In his book *Inside the New Age Nightmare,* he writes, "What used to be as obvious as an orange robed Hare Krishna devotee or a blissed out

Hippie would come today as a man in a three-piece suit or laboratory coat."[1] Or, we might add, a Bible quoting evangelist. Educators, research scientists, doctors, nurses, ministers—everyone, it seems, is becoming involved in healing. No wonder we are confused.

So what can we do? Whom can we trust?

RED FLAGS TO WATCH FOR

The following thirteen red flags can help you tell when you may be in danger of crossing the line from the helpful practitioner to the harmful.

Red Flag No. 1: An Unscientific Approach

Ask yourself: Is this therapy within the scientific mainstream? If its founders cannot get their findings published in such well respected scientific journals such as *The Journal of the American Medical Association* or *The New England Journal of Medicine,* you should suspect something is wrong.

Next ask yourself, Who is pushing the therapy? Is it someone who stands to benefit personally? The National Health Federation (NHF), for instance, is one group that promotes unproven cancer therapies. How is the practitioner or the organization he represents financed? The National Health Federation is financed primarily through membership fees and donations, and through advertising revenue from its publication *Health Freedom News*. Sixty percent of the periodical's contents is advertising for questionable products, devices, and mail-order courses in homeopathy, naturopathy, reflexology, iridology, toxicity testing, herbal products, and the services available from "clinics" across the border in Mexico, according to *CA—A Cancer Journal for Clinicians* (Jan/Feb 1991).

Then there are groups that sound as if they are looking out for the consumer's interest, like the Council for Responsible Nutrition. But the Council is in fact a Washington, D.C., group which represents manufacturers and distributors of food supplements sold through health food stores. Hardly a disinterested party.

How can you avoid being tricked by clever promoters? It's not always easy. But inquiring at a reputable source of medical information such as the American Cancer Society is a good place to start.

Red Flag No. 2: Claims to Manipulate Energy or Use Psychic Power

Elements of the melding of folklore and fact were prevalent up until the last 150 years of medical history. To a degree some blending still exists today, like a mom's propensity to put an aromatic ointment on her sick child's chest. Why? No reason, except that it harks back to the days when physicians were scarce and mothers would lovingly apply poultices to their children's chests in an attempt to ease the little ones' discomfort.

Yet with the development of scientific methods and improved research skills, the pendulum of scientific opinion swung clearly away from the supernatural. Practitioners associated with various groups and organizations now fill this spiritual void in the practice of medicine. Extreme caution, however, must be used before consulting them.

For instance, an organization called Metaphysicians, founded in 1985 by San Francisco Bay area physician Terry Tyler, counts over 100 doctors in its membership. According to Tyler, this is the first known group of medical doctors who are "as apt to invoke the help of spirits, or the energy of the universe, as they are to prescribe an antibiotic."[2]

Dr. Tyler describes his fellow metaphysicians as being "physicians with a spiritual sense." What this means, he says, is that they are "one with everything," that they see every living and non-living thing in the world as a part of the same "seamless web of energy, and thus related in the most intimate way." (Note the New Age philosophy.)

Tyler claims that this style of medicine is "backed by good

science," a statement many in the medical world—ourselves included—would strongly contest. He may be a medical doctor graduated from a prestigious university, but his claims of energy and psychic power cause the red flags to fly high, both from a scientific and a Christian perspective.

Red Flag No. 3: Attempts to Make You Alone or the 'Power Within' Responsible for Your Health

Watch out for a practitioner who insists it is the placebo response of your own "inner physician" that heals you. Ask yourself, If my inner response does in fact heal me, why do I need this practitioner in the first place?

A holistic practitioner who is also a medical doctor answered a reader's question on how to choose an alternative M.D. in *East-West* magazine, June 1986. His advice was to find one who would support "the healer within." People considering this, he wrote, should see how they wish to promote optimum health for themselves.

It makes me wonder what kind of advice a patient can depend on if all he has in a physician is a "yes man" obeying the whims of the "power within" each patient—Yes to this, Yes to that, Yes to anything the patient wants to do or to try, regardless of the validity of the method.

Where are the Bernie Siegels, the Kübler-Rosses and the Gerald Jampolskis when it comes to speaking out against the indisputable evidence of potential harm and ineffectiveness of many of today's popular alternative therapies? They are standing back in the shadows reluctant to take a stand for truth. Bernie Siegel wants us to use "meditative and life-style-altering techniques . . . to gain access to the superintelligence" he says resides within each of us.[3] He equates this superintelligence with God, Self, life force, or DNA. Would this "superintelligence" approve of a cancer patient using methods such as Laetrile which have been proven worthless and harmful? Referring to Laetrile he asserts that if the patient's belief system enables it to work, he is certainly not going to use the authority of his profession to destroy its benefits. Perhaps we need to remind Bernie of the Latin phrase known to all physicians: *Primum non nocere*—first do no harm.

Red Flag No. 4: Other Authorities Aren't Familiar with the Therapy

Alternative health practitioner Adelle Davis used to say she never saw anyone get cancer who drank a quart of milk a day as she did. Her books, such as *Let's Get Well* and *Let's Have Healthy Children* have sold millions, and large numbers of them continue to sell today. In 1974 Adelle Davis died of cancer.

Davis promoted hundreds of unfounded nutritional theories, including the concept that crib death could be prevented by breast feeding plus adding vitamin E to the baby's diet. She was opposed to the pasteurization of milk. Frequently she recommended high doses of vitamins A and D.

Adelle Davis was hailed by the public as a pioneer in the world of nutritional therapy. Unfortunately for some of her followers, adherence to her dietary regimens resulted in serious harm. An out-of-court settlement for $150,000 was won against her estate and the publisher of her book *Let's Have Healthy Children* because a little girl's nervous system was permanently damaged when her parents gave her toxic doses of vitamin A as recommended in the book. For at least one baby, the consequences were deadly. An infant in Florida died from high doses of potassium advised in the book.[4]

Many alternative health quacks proclaim miraculous breakthroughs. But their methods have several qualities in common: (1) They have not been subjected to acceptable proof of their effectiveness. (2) Proponents have no idea why the method works. "It just works," they explain. (3) Most often they discount the need for controlled tests, preferring to rely on the biased testimonials of a few selected patients.

Sometimes a medical breakthrough really does occur. When this happens, you can be sure it won't be kept a secret. It will be used by physicians across the country and widely discussed in newspapers, magazines, and on television.

Red Flag No. 5: Claims That the Therapy Is a Cure-all

Sometimes alternative practitioners use what has been described as "simpleton science." They argue that all disease has but one cause, so one treatment is all that is needed to fight it. We can see an example of this thinking in the statement: "Bad nutrition causes all disease, therefore good nutrition cures it."

Magazine articles and advertisements for these "cure-all" products are usually carefully written to include a disclaimer. After all, advertisers don't want to be held liable for false advertising. Yet in the text of the magazine they often make blatant claims. Under the protection of freedom of the press they misquote, exaggerate, and in many cases outright lie about the extraordinary results of particular treatments.

Scientific medicine emphasizes accurate and precise diagnosis before beginning treatment, so that appropriate therapy can be prescribed. Alternative medical practitioners, on the other hand, are not particularly concerned about an exact diagnosis. They are much more willing to accept this "one treatment fits all" approach.

Red Flag No. 6: Claims of Extraordinary Cure Rates

Be extremely cautious of anyone claiming 100 or 90 percent success rates. Also watch out for anyone who claims a cure that is totally safe and without side effects.

Practitioners in clinics in Tijuana, Mexico, promoted by Americans, claim not only to be able to detect cancer but also to find pre-cancerous conditions. While there are certain well established pre-cancer conditions such as colon polyps which often become malignant, the bogus clinics are claiming to ward off cancer in completely healthy individuals, people who are simply worried about developing cancer sometime.

Besides cancer, these so-called clinics claim to have cures for such conditions as arthritis and multiple sclerosis. The director at one Tijuana clinic has openly stated that there are indeed known causes and cures for these very diseases, despite the fact that leading medical scientists have many, many questions about them.

When a patient arrives at such a clinic, many bogus tests are performed, such as blood crystallization, live cell analysis, iridology (diagnosis by examining the iris of the eye) and applied kinesiology (muscle testing). Treatments at the clinics typically include special diets with up to 300 supplements a day; glandular tissue extract; enzyme therapies; spiritual and faith healing—often including psychic surgery and detoxification, which consists of a heavily vegetarian diet followed by colonics such as coffee enemas.

These clinics often have their own brand of metabolic therapy. Following a diagnosis—most likely achieved through either iridology or applied kinesiology—the patient goes through a process of detoxification by fasting or enemas. This is followed by the building up of the patient's immune system by food supplement. Treatments are unconventional to say the least. At one clinic, practitioners take a blood sample from a patient's neck, treat the sample with 500 volts of direct electricity, then transfuse it back into the patient. At another, hydrogen peroxide is injected into the blood to increase oxygen and supposedly kill cancer cells. Unfortunately, treatments such as these are also taking place throughout America.

Dr. James Lowell, vice president of the National Council Against Health Fraud, states that the worst of the Tijuana clinics doesn't even have running water.[5] Even so, it is reported to gross more than $100,000 a month. Patients, it seems, just can't resist the promise of a cure.

Some of my AIDS and cancer patients have died, but others are still alive. As yet we can't cure all forms of cancer, and certainly not AIDS. We can, however, prolong the lives of many sufferers. Only quacks claim to have cures for everything.

Red Flag No. 7: Warnings of a 'Medical Conspiracy'

After Mary Ann (the woman in a preceding chapter who left her family for treatment in Mexico) was diagnosed as having cancer, acquaintances came over to her house with a video they said would open up a whole new arena of possibilities. The message of the video was a denunciation of what they termed an American Medical Association (AMA) conspiracy. They have a cure for cancer, the video stated, but they're hiding it. It is to their financial advantage to keep patients coming back. The claims disgusted Mary Ann's husband. Not Mary Ann. She bought it all.

Conspiracy claims do drive people to alternative health practitioners. Sometimes the supposed conspiracy is laid at the feet of the Federal Drug Administration. Other times it's the fault of the AMA or other established medical groups. Whoever is to blame, the idea is the same: Governmental or medical conspirators are depriving people of their chances for good health.

Let's think about this for a minute. A conspiracy of this magnitude would have to include all elements of the medical profession, from medical schools to scientific researchers to individual physicians. The supposed reasoning is this: If doctors can keep people sick by preventing them from learning to heal themselves, then somehow the medical community, pharmaceutical companies, and the government itself will benefit. Paranoid thinking? You bet! Yet many people accept it. Just look at Laetrile's success.

Many alternative health practitioners liken themselves to misunderstood scientists destined to be the heroes of the future. Like Galileo, they say, they are misunderstood by blind and closed-minded scientists.

Red Flag No. 8: The Practitioner's Explanations Don't Make Sense

We in the health profession have an obligation to provide accurate health information to our patients. And certainly it's appropriate for our patients to demand accurate, scientifically based, factual information with regards to their medical care.

Any time a practitioner prescribes something that seems off the wall, you should ask questions: How do you know that? How can you be sure? What does it mean? If the answers come only in vague terms, beware. The person to whom you're talking, the book you're reading, or the information source you're consulting may not know what they're talking about.

Frequently alternative health osteopathics exploit the fear of illness and death that lies within all of us, especially the fear of patients who have incurable illnesses or chronic pain. The promise of painless treatment and guaranteed results is hard for anyone to ignore. An example of this is the practitioner who proposes a metabolic diet cure for his cancer patient instead of chemotherapy. "Chemotherapy is poison," he tells her. "It will kill you."

Dr. John Renner, president of the Midwest Council on Health Fraud, went up to a clerk at a health food store in Lansing, Michigan, and asked, "Do you have anything that will keep me from getting AIDS?" He was sold a bottle of herbal septic.

Since the bottle label states that this product is a topical and oral germ killer and infection fighter, Dr. Renner asked the clerk how he was to use it.

"Well," he was told, "you could gargle with it or you could, you know, wipe it on your skin." That was as precise as the instructions got.

The advice found in books on alternative medicine range from the unlikely to the downright ludicrous. One suggestion in *Curing AIDS Now* suggests exposing the genitals to the sunlight at 4 P.M. at a forty-five-degree angle. Crystal therapy is very big in AIDS prevention. You can buy flower petals for aroma therapy, and endless books on how to pump up your immune system through soup, vitamins, herbal therapies, homeopathic therapy, and mental therapy such as thinking positively. A tabloid newspaper recently told of an AIDS victim in a remote village in France who was supposedly cured by alien beings on a spaceship that landed and took the sick man on board.

The most incredible stories and explanations are accepted by some people—usually the most desperate among us.

Red Flag No. 9: The Practitioner's Qualifications Are Questionable

Jane Fonda has reportedly been given acupuncture treatments by a Brazilian veterinarian who specializes in treating horses. He began by treating Fonda's horses. Two years later he was treating her.

The interaction between a patient and her practitioner is seen quite differently in alternative medicine. Alternative practitioners view their relationship with their patients as one of equal partners, since it doesn't require extensive training to become a practitioner. In fact, they often operate as resources for their patients rather than as authoritarian figures.

Consider Carlton Fredricks, Ph.D., a well-known nutritionist and columnist for *Prevention* magazine's "Hotline to Health."

He has virtually no training in any health science; he graduated from the University of Alabama with a major in English and a minor in political science. The City Magistrates Court of New York indicates that Fredricks was charged with practicing medicine without a license and fined after pleading guilty to diagnosing patients and prescribing vitamins for their illnesses. The alternative health movement is charging unfair harassment of a pioneer in the nutritional field.[6]

Fredricks received his Ph.D. in communications; he never took a single course in nutrition. Yet as one of the originators of the crusade to discredit sugar, he was presented on the Merv Griffin and Johnny Carson shows as a "leading nutritional consultant."

The problem is, unqualified practitioners can look extremely professional. They are usually smooth and articulate. They often have a variety of degrees framed and hanging on their walls. Credentials, however, can come from many different sources. Diploma mills are easy to locate. Credentials can even be ordered through mail-order catalogues. In many cases, a person's participation in an organization in no way implies either competency or expertise in his field.

Victor Herbert, a physician and national expert on health fraud, says many of today's nutrition snake-oil salespeople are members of the American Association of Nutrition Consultants. Membership in this association, one that gives a beautiful diploma with its own gold seal and red ribbons, appears impressive indeed. The diploma says that the named person "is a professional member of a professional association dedicated to maintaining ethical standards in nutrition and dietary consulting." What it doesn't say is that its promoters are actively working to prevent consumer protection laws, which would license real nutritionists and dietitians in various states.[7]

To document how blatant the deception is, Dr. Herbert says there are only three criteria for obtaining this credential:

(1) You must have a name, as it will be inscribed on the document.

(2) You must have an address so the document can be mailed to you.

(3) You must have a check for $50 to accompany your application.[8]

How does he know these are the only requirements? His dog, Sassafrass, is a professional member of the American Association of Nutrition!

Currently there are 25,000 people in the United States with this credential. (We don't know how many dogs.) The organization even publishes a magazine called *Nutrition Consultant*. Most likely, it's available in your local health food store.

(Evidently Dr. Herbert's cat, Charley, was upset that Sassafrass was a nutrition consultant. To placate him, Dr. Herbert decided to invest $50 so Charley could become a member of the even more prestigious International Academy of Nutritional Consultants. Unfortunately for Charley, his organization merged into Sassafrass's organization, so now they both belong to the American Association of Nutrition Consultants.)

When David sent for information from the American Holistic

College of Nutrition—which is high on our list of questionable organizations—he received a postcard invitation to work toward a B.S., M.S., or doctoral degree in nutrition from their college, located in Birmingham, Alabama. After taking the courses of study, the postcard said, he would be able to set up his nutritional counseling practice, both profitably and legally. And if he were to enroll within thirty days, he would receive a 15 percent reduction in his tuition.

We had our office manager call the 800 number and inquire about the prerequisites for entering their program. "I don't have a college degree," she explained. She was assured, "That's not necessary for the B.S. degree. You must have a B.S. degree, however, to enter the master's program and both a college and a master's degree to enter the doctoral program. . . . This can be easily accomplished," the representative assured her. "The cost for all three classes, the B.S., the M.S., and the Ph.D., is only $1,850. If paid in advance, $1,480."

There's more. The whole process takes only fourteen months and is all reading. The tests are sent in by mail. For the master's degree, a 2,000-word dissertation on a subject of your choosing is required.

Is this legal? Absolutely—as long as the graduate bills herself as a consultant rather than as a physician.

How does a consultant practice? Well, my manager was told the typical procedure is to have a patient fill out a questionnaire, and from that she would know what was wrong with the person. She would use such words as "suggest" and "recommend" treatment. That would keep her from crossing into the area of prescribing or diagnosing.

"Has anyone ever failed these courses?" my office manager asked.

"No, no one," was the cheery reply. "In fact, there's a money back guarantee within thirty days if you're not completely satisfied."

The eleven-by-fourteen-inch diploma she would receive would read: American College of Nutrition, Bachelor of Science (or Master of Science, or Doctor of Philosophy) from Birmingham, Alabama. It would be signed by Dr. Clayton, the institution president, and would, we're sure, be suitable for framing.

"As a consultant, your fee would be 50 to 75 dollars per session," my manager was assured. She was told about one graduate who finished her course in just two months and was now practicing in a chiropractor's office. "Another finished in three months," the college representative explained.

Before you put too much credence in an organization or the initials behind a name ask: What are this organization's membership requirements? Does it require any scientific expertise, or just a willingness to pay dues?

The mere fact that an individual belongs to an organization or has several initials behind her name should not impress you in the least.

Red Flag No. 10: Primary Proof Is from Testimonials

Often the testimonials of the "cured" lure people into a technique or a specific product. But look cautiously at therapies that rely heavily on testimonials and stories. Are the sources proven and reputable? Might they be biased?

Health anecdotes and testimonials in general are worthless as evidence of either the safety or the efficacy of a product. To be valid, remedies must be verified by responsible health professionals. The supposed effect may have occurred by coincidence, by suggestion, by a misunderstanding, or even by outright falsehood. In many cases the patients believed they had a disease they never had at all.

In order to accept a claimed cure as valid, Dr. Herbert, the expert on fraud, outlines four necessary conditions:

First, the patient must actually have the disease. That is, the condition must be established by responsible criteria.

Second, the claimed cure must result from the therapy. If a therapy is only promoted through the tight-knit world of alternative medicine, with no objective proof of efficacy from reputable scientific observers, it is usually not just questionable but probably downright false. Even if there is an improvement in one's health after using the therapy, it doesn't necessarily follow that the treatment itself had anything to do with the improvement—other factors could have been at work.

Third, the disease must, in fact, be cured rather than merely progressing without symptoms. This can be documented by x-ray, lab tests, biopsy, or a physician's examination.

Fourth, the patient must be alive. That is, he must have survived the treatment.[9]

Before you put much stock in a testimonial, make sure it is valid.

Red Flag No. 11: Heavy Reliance on Altered States of Consciousness

Any practice which promotes a state of altered consciousness—meditation, yoga, Transcendental Meditation, visualization, hypnosis, or shamanic trance—should cause you concern. This is a staple in many areas of alternative health care, especially those with an occultic influence.

Under carefully defined and proper methods, there may be limited opportunities for using an altered state of consciousness in the legitimate area of hypnosis. In general, however, anyone who doesn't want her mind to be manipulated should avoid such a state.

Red Flag No. 12: Christian Language or Endorsements to Guarantee Legitimacy

A large dose of spiritual concepts and Christian principles is often mixed in with questionable health methods and remedies. I have a business card from a man who calls himself a Christian channeler. He claims to provide information for people on their health and well-being by channeling spirit guides in a "Christian manner." Because he calls himself a Christian, it is possible that some people may lower their guard and more readily accept his advice. Such unscrupulous individuals abound within the alternative health movement, quoting the Bible and Jesus, all the while promoting fraud and deception.

A pastor in Pennsylvania tells of an elder on his board who was into homeopathic medicine. The elder got two other people in the church started on it as well as a man from another church. Everyone involved swore the homeopathic remedies worked, and they praised God for allowing His Holy Spirit to accomplish His work.

When the pastor approached the elder with his concerns, the man really listened and did some serious thinking. "He didn't want to take a chance on anything that could be linked to the enemy," the pastor told me. In the end the elder threw out all the homeopathic medicines. Then he spoke to the others about the errors in the therapy's philosophy.

Sometimes it's the pastor who perpetrates the deception. From his position of authority, covered by the convictions that Christians wouldn't lie and that pastors are privy to special insights, it isn't difficult for them to draw others into their alternative health practices.

A nice brochure sent out by the New England Health Center in Boston, Massachusetts, might cause Christians to believe it is a Christian-oriented organization. An insert in the brochure features Psalm 139. Actually, the founder of this health center is a naturopath who uses such questionable techniques as homeopathy, herbal therapy, and the energy manipulating system of acupuncture. The group advertises that it is beginning a meditation and spiritual reading group. But meditation doesn't always mean prayer as we know it, and spiritual doesn't always mean biblical Christianity.

I received a brochure in the mail the other day from an institute of Holistic Theology, offering mail-order doctorates of divinity for alternative healers. If you pay in advance, you can receive a degree that gives you the freedom to practice holistic health based on principles the institutes often claim are found in the Bible. The degree protects the alternative healers under the Constitution's guarantee of "freedom of religion," though their practices are questionable. The promotion of fraud under the guise of religion is one of the cruelest hoaxes of all and should be vigorously opposed by all within the church.

References, testimonials, or endorsements from religious figures don't guarantee legitimacy, either. Whether doctor, pastor, speaker, author, or celebrity, don't allow anyone to lead you astray.

Red Flag No. 13: Claims that Reduce the Practitioner's Accountability

A former naturopathic doctor himself, Randall Baer says, "I see this field as being a mixture of positive and negative. Three ingredients of wholesome and six ingredients of New Age. Nine ingredients of healthy and twenty of the New Age. In this tricky, subtle, holistic health field, discernment is at a premium." He adds, "From my own experience, over seventy percent of holistic health professionals have an underlying New Age based philosophy."[10]

That's interesting. Especially since many practitioners with New Age roots are careful not to advertise the fact.

Roger Miller, editor of the *FDA Consumer,* wrote an article entitled "The Voice of the Quack." In it he states that language is one of the ways to help identify questionable practitioners. Such language is often mystical. Today's practitioner is likely to evoke scientific sounding terminology such as "an amazing breakthrough in medical technology" or "clinical studies prove that . . ." or "researchers have uncovered the secret that revolutionizes the science of . . ." When you hear such statements from practitioners, view them with skepticism.

Other statements to watch out for include: "Now from Europe comes a remarkable breakthrough in . . ." and "100 percent natural. Works safely and naturally." Beware of testimonial language such as "it really works," and practices which allude to secret formulas. Be wary when you read advertisements that promote breakthroughs: "secret formula," "instant cures," "100 percent safe," "100 percent painless."

In the end, practitioners who offer therapies that are unsound, dangerous, or deceptive *are accountable to their patients*. The right to take people's money by deceit and endanger their health is not a right at all. But if you and I don't hold them accountable, who will? It's the responsibility of each of us to hold therapists responsible. We must refuse to be tricked. We need to know the red flags and we must watch for them.

Later in this book, we will look at the alternative health care methods in four categories—natural therapies, mind therapies, energy manipulating therapies, and supernatural therapies— and expose the myths that often creep into this care. We all know that an educated consumer is a wise consumer. When we are talking about health care, an educated consumer is also a healthy, alive consumer!

Chapter Five

IT'S NATURAL, BUT IS IT REALLY BETTER?

Natural Therapies

Picture Sylvia: overweight, pale, sickly, aching joints. Every month she suffered flu symptoms and yeast infections. Some days she felt so bad she couldn't get out of bed. Each day she grew more depressed. And she was angry. Why couldn't the doctors cure her?

"This had been going on for three years," Sylvia said. "I was getting desperate."

It was a naturopath, Sylvia says, who finally offered her help. He told Sylvia that she was allergic to many foods. He also said she was suffering from chronic mononucleosis. It was this diagnosis that began Sylvia's diligent search for health alternatives. Mainly she turned to herbs and eating healthy foods.

Today Sylvia, who calls herself a "certified natural health counselor," offers individual counseling in her home. She also teaches iridology, a method she describes as a study of the iris of the eye which can reveal weaknesses within the body. And she evaluates a person's health by muscle testing. "The strength or weakness of various muscles can show much about the condition of organs, glands, and nerves," she claims.

Still, Sylvia insists she neither diagnoses diseases nor prescribes medicines. "I am merely educating the person as to the

78

origin of their health problems according to analysis of the weak areas of their body,'' she says. Yet she goes on to state that she has found that the proper use of herbs can be a key to rebuilding the body's weak areas.

It's always wonderful to hear of a person who has found a solution to her suffering. Certainly there are many who, like Sylvia, suffer from conditions which are often difficult to diagnose and treat. They, too, get frustrated when, despite doctors' testings and probings and evaluations, neither diagnosis nor cure is forthcoming.

Yet while we can be happy that Sylvia feels better, we have to stop and ask: Just how accurate is the information in her story? (It appeared in the Neighborhood section of a North Carolina newspaper.) Her symptoms sound similar to those of chronic fatigue syndrome, an as yet poorly understood chronic debilitating illness. What is clearly understood is that the practices described are totally without scientific validity. Sylvia's statement that the ''iris is an extension of the brain'' is an anatomical impossibility. And her credentials as a natural health counselor? She was trained in a multilevel marketing organization for herbs and vitamins whose primary motive was profit. Two red flags here—unscientific treatments practiced by a person with questionable qualifications.

Who are the practitioners who turn to nature and natural products as the true healers of the afflictions of humankind? Let's identify them and explore what they purport to do.

AYURVEDA

Ayurveda has been getting a lot of press lately. The following is from a question/answer article in the Who's Who column in our local newspaper:

Q: How does Margaret Thatcher retain her girlish figure and trampoline-taut skin at 62?
A: For the rejuvention of the aging body and skin, Thatcher has relied in recent years on a certain Indian woman in Britain who

practices the ancient health system of Ayurveda. After paying $1,000, Thatcher disrobes and lowers herself into a tub filled with Italian mud. The viscous liquid is then charged with .3 amps of electricity which recharges her nervous system and releases blocked energy. After washing up and popping a pill of royal bee jelly, another of her beauty secrets, she is refreshed and ready to take on the world which she often does.[1]

Interesting picture. Notice the references to manipulating energy? Another red flag.

Yet if a great woman like Margaret Thatcher submits to Ayurveda, certainly there must be something to it. At the very least, it must be a harmless practice. One would think so. But read on.

What Is Ayurveda?

Ayurveda is an out and out promotion of spiritual concepts. This ancient folk medicine from India claims to incorporate the concepts of medicine, psychology, culture, religion, and philosophy into one grab bag of health care. It came directly from ancient Hindus who, through religious practice and meditation or an altered state of consciousness, came up with this so-called "scientific" method of healing. (Another red flag!)

Ayurveda consists of massages, herbal baths, meditation, and long walks. Not bad so far. Supposedly it works through positive emotions, body awareness, and mental detachment from illness. Therapists credit Ayurveda with subduing such problems as chronic migraine headaches and with eliminating pains that have no identifiable cause. They claim it even brings cancer into remission—although Dr. Deepak Chopra, an endocrinologist who runs his own Ayurveda clinic, says that when someone quickly improves or overcomes a chronic illness thru Ayurveda therapy, that person has merely triggerd his body's own healing response and cured the condition.

Ayurveda comes from a Hindu word meaning the science or

knowledge of life. Its basic tenet is that the mind and body are not separate entities. They are one and the same. According to Chopra, every single cell in each part of the body, from the liver to the kidneys to the heart, has its own mind. Chopra insists a person can achieve a mind/body balance through the activities his clinic offers. What are these activities? Well, a treatment designed to "profoundly relax the nervous system" involves the slow pouring of sesame oil onto the patient's forehead.

Still More Red Flags

Says Chopra, "As soon as you lose your attachment to your disease, the sooner the disease also seems to go away." How's that for creating your own reality? It's your responsibility: do you choose to have your disease, or do you not? Make up your mind! (Red Flag No. 3.)

Chopra is eager to claim 100 percent cure rates for some disorders, such as mild hypertension and migraine headaches. Not even the most experienced physician would dare make such a claim. For more serious disorders, including coronary artery disease, he claims Ayurveda practitioners are able to free as many as 50 to 60 percent of their patients of the symptoms. (Red Flag No. 6.) Though he says he cooperates with his patients' other therapies, such as chemotherapy, his tendency is to move away from such treatments.

"I frequently see patients taking therapies that are really distressing," he said, "for example, patients with lung cancer who are getting radiation or chemotherapy which isn't doing anything but destroying the patients."[2] He is apparently oblivious to the fact that these very therapies are verifiably proven helpful in many cases.

The charismatic figure behind Ayurveda is Maharishi Yogi, the founder of the Transcendental Meditation movement. Dr. Chopra recognizes that he is a disciple of the Yogi, whom he describes as "one of the greatest living sages." For his part, the Maharishi considers Ayurveda so beneficial that it is a major factor in his global campaign to create a disease-free society in every country. He has singled Chopra out to deliver the special Ayurveda techniques to the West. Once again we see the intense Eastern, or New Age, religious emphasis, this time disguised as "nouveau medicine" for the rich and famous.

The cost of a consultation with an Ayurveda physician does not come cheap—$145 for the initial visit and $75 for subsequent evaluations at Chopra's Pacific Palisades Center. According to Chopra, insurance companies now reimburse Ayurveda patients for their treatments. That's not too surprising. Even though the therapies are highly questionable, the practitioners are licensed physicians. Even within mainstream medicine, the Ayurveda movement is picking up speed and interest.

A recent article advocating Ayurveda appeared in the *Journal of the American Medical Association* (265:2636–7, 1991), alleging that "a growing number of Western physicians . . . are finding it to add valuable knowledge that is complementary to modern allopathic medicine." What the article didn't say was that Ayur-Veda™ is a trade name for a line of health foods and medical services headed by the Maharishi Mehesh Yogi, guru of the TM movement. Apparently the Maharishi has named Deepak Chopra, M.D., who was one of the *JAMA* article authors, "Dhanvantari (Lord of Immortality) the keeper of perfect health for the world." As a chief promoter of Ayur-Veda™, Chopra is not exactly an unbiased observer.

Now, we're not arguing with the Ayurveda slogan, "sound body, sound mind." And some of the therapies, including a low fat diet, would be good for any of us. The problem is that there is another side to the slogan. If we accept the idea that positive thinking can cure an illness, we have to accept also that if one isn't cured, that person must have had negative thoughts. Sick people suffer enough misery from their illnesses. They shouldn't also be made to bear the blame for having the illness. That would be cruel enough if it were a proven fact. That it's nothing more than a flimsy and totally unsubstantiated theory makes it all the worse.

BODYWORK

Bodywork is not a single technique. It refers to many procedures. Those who practice bodywork believe people can profoundly influence their physical and emotional well-being by using hands to rid the body of chronic muscular tension. This is the core of all bodywork disciplines.

Even the noted alternative health book *Positive Living and Health,* which has definite New Age leanings, offers a word of warning in the front of the section on bodywork: "The real challenge is to separate what is half-baked from what is legitimate and determine which of the reputable methods is most likely to offer you what you need."

Indeed, this is the problem we face when we look at the bodywork techniques. Certainly it is vital that we learn to differentiate between what is legitimate and what is "half-baked." But our challenge goes even deeper. We need to consider the spiritual aspects of each therapy as well as the spiritual inclinations of those espousing them.

Massage Therapy

We're not talking about massage parlors here, not those sexually oriented establishments we associate with seedy buildings on the outskirts of town. What we're talking about is the physical work of the hands working on the body's tissues for medical purposes.

The problem with massage therapy is that in many cases it seems to have overstepped the bounds of simply working on the tissues of the body, and moved into the arena of mind/body linkage. In other words, by working on the tissues of the body, practitioners think they can impact the mind as well.

Most of us would agree that it feels good to have someone touch us. The hands-on therapy of massage therapists may meet this very real need human beings have to be touched by others. And with dimmed lights and a skilled masseuse, relaxation will no doubt occur. But when one undergoes massage therapy, is it possible that he is being touched in other ways? Is he simply getting a massage for his stiff, sore muscles, or can the massage therapist actually delve into his subconscious?

I know, I know. This all sounds a bit far-fetched. But let me give you an example. When I first entered medical practice, a massage therapist asked to come and speak with me in my office. She was hoping to get referrals. This young lady began by explaining her techniques. Then she told me the ways in which she felt her practice would be compatible and helpful to my patients who suffered from chronic pain or injuries such as whiplash and low back strains. That all sounded fine. But the next thing she said was that she sometimes did special massages with a spiritual aspect.

"Spiritual aspect?" I asked.

"Out-of-body experiences," she explained. "Sometimes my patients are able to have them."

A bit alarmed, I told her, "That has nothing to do with what you were trained for and are licensed to practice."

The lady disagreed—loudly and forcefully. "Narrow-minded" is one of the ways she described me. We parted on a bitterly strained note. Needless to say, she got no referrals from me.

Certainly not all massage therapists work this way. Yet this philosophy does pervade current massage therapy.

Massage therapists associated with the American Massage Therapy Association are not poorly trained. Their required program consists of at least 500 classroom hours of training.

Yet questionable practices are embraced by some schools of massage therapy. In addition to anatomy, physiology, and traditional massage courses, they offer such courses as reflexology (we will hear more about this later) and polarity therapy, an energy balancing technique. One school licensed by the state of New Hampshire has on staff a chiropractor who lists as his credits expertise in iridology, nutrition (non-traditional), herbology, homeopathy, and chiropractic. I don't know about you, but I would have to question the legitimacy of this school based on the credentials of this staff member alone since we know that iridology has no scientific basis. And, as far as the nutrition goes, few chiropractors talk about the same things Sharon does in her private nutrition practice and their training does not even compare to Sharon's. She studied nutrition for four years, has her Ph.D. in nutrition, and is a registered dietitian, whereas many of the chiropractors have taken a few hours of lectures from dubious instructors at best.

When we look at individual massage therapists, it's difficult to know whether or not we will be influenced by some of their practices. What we do know is that many of the therapists graduating and practicing today are heavily influenced by the alternative health movement. Some are convinced these techniques should be wholeheartedly embraced. Even so, massage therapy is probably the most legitimate of all the bodywork therapies.

Rolfing

Rolfing is similar in some ways to massage therapy, but there is a big difference between the two. Rolfing consists of a series of ten basic bodywork sessions which are said to be "deep connective tissue manipulation."

This technique was named after its founder, Ida P. Rolf, who called her system Structural Integration. The supposed aim of rolfing is to increase muscular length and overall balance for optimal posture. That rolfing is simply a variant on the metaphysical healing theory of energy manipulation is clear by Rolf's own words. She described her system as an attempt to "realign the random body into an orderly, balanced energy system that can operate in the field of gravity."[3]

In 1916, Rolf, who had a Ph.D. in biochemistry from Columbia University's College of Physicians and Surgeons, became interested in bodywork and body mechanics through an initial practice of yoga. It seems that Rolf explored many different manipulative therapies before finally inventing her own approach. She saw her methods as a unified systematic approach to healing and reported changes in her subjects' "energy bodies," which were confirmed by an "aura reader."

Aside from that far-out basis of care, the theory behind rolfing sounds pretty good. It holds that the force of gravity and poor posture combine to throw the body out of proper alignment. As a result, certain muscles are thrown into an unnatural contraction. As the muscle builds up, the connective tissues develop in the body and other problems can follow: Joints lose their freedom and circulation is restricted. But that's just the beginning. According to rolfing theory, pain, anger, and other emotional states are repressed and held in this tense musculature.

Unlike other energy manipulations, rolfing simply seeks to align the body so as to allow the force of gravity to perform its work. The only area that seems to be a potential problem is rolfers' real goal of releasing memories and emotions from their clients during rolfing sessions. Rolf believed that the techniques of deep tissue massage, which in many cases are quite painful, may actually be able to relieve a lifelong buildup of muscular "armoring." This armoring is said to be a way we build a bodily barrier for all our physical and psychic wounds in life.

Trager Work

Trager work is a body-mind procedure created by Elton Trager. It is a combination of hands-on and movement techniques practiced in a relaxed, meditative state Trager calls "the hookup."

Trager, who received an M.D. degree from the medical school in Guadalajara, Mexico, has practiced in Hawaii for more than twenty years. His aim in trager work is to break up neuro-muscular holdings that supposedly develop in response to accidents, illnesses, and emotional trauma. It's sort of the culmination of all the physical baggage one might accumulate during life. Trager workers see patterns of restrictive stiffness, tension, and pain as products of an unconscious mental process. A key concept here is that the body and mind are inseparable. The focus of Trager's work becomes "mind to mind" communication between the practitioner and his client.

The intention of tragering, then, is to allow the patient to give up conscious muscular control and drift into a deeply relaxed state. "The hookup" is the key to this communication between the practitioner and the patient. During the one and one-half-hour sessions, the therapist cradles the client in his arms while he guides her passive body in a series of gentle movements. When the hookup is achieved, there is supposedly some sort of mental give and take that takes place from the practitioner to the client.

Both the client and the therapist are expected to enter meditative, or altered, states of consciousness (red flag!). The therapist empties his mind of all thoughts and feelings, except for a sense of how light and free the body can feel. It is this thought of light and free body motion that is communicated through the therapist's massage techniques to the client.

Trager work primarily focuses on severe neuro-muscular disturbances that do not respond well to typical conventional therapy—victims of such diseases as polio, multiple sclerosis, and muscular dystrophy. Trager does advise caution in working with cancer and other diseases he feels need to be treated by other means. It is not coincidental that many alternative therapies are directed towards problems which are difficult to diagnose and to treat.

A major problem with trager work is its use of meditation within an altered state of consciousness. Any time a person submits to such a state, there is the danger of mental suggestibility, and an entry way for spiritual problems for which the patient never bargained.

CHIROPRACTIC MEDICINE

There are more than 30,000 chiropractors licensed to practice in the United States. In one year (1984), 163 million office visits were made to them. Most likely only a very small number of their patients realize that many chiropractors do not maintain the same view of health and disease held by medical scientists worldwide.

Perhaps even more disturbing is the increasingly whole-hearted acceptance of unscientific New Age medical practices by the chiropractic community. Once again, a popular and easily accessed area of health care leads unsuspecting patients into highly questionable and deceptive practices.

During a particularly pressure-filled time in her life, Dottie began suffering headaches.

"The problem is in your spine," her chiropractor told her.

Although Dottie had little money—she worked for $4 an hour cleaning houses—he said she needed treatments twice a week. When her headaches decreased, he said she still needed the treatments—indefinitely. "Maintenance," he explained.

Steve was in a car accident in which he fractured his leg. When he continued to limp, he consulted a chiropractor who prescribed weekly treatments. His limp didn't improve. He was told to come in twice a week. When Steve finally consulted a neurologist, his condition was diagnosed as genetic nerve degeneration. No amount of manipulation could keep his condition from worsening.

What Is Chiropractic Medicine?

Good question. You've heard of chiropractors. Many of you have been treated by one. You call him Doctor, and your insurance likely paid his bill. He adjusted your back. Perhaps he sold you vitamins. But just what is a chiropractor?

A wide variation of practitioners is gathered under the umbrella term chiropractor. Some offer straight manipulative practices. Many mix in other types of treatments. Some drift into questionable alternative care practices.

Chiropractic medicine wasn't founded by a physician at all, but by Daniel David Palmer, a traveling merchant. He began his lay healing practice in 1886, after claiming to have miraculously restored the hearing of a deaf janitor who worked in his building by simply adjusting the man's neck. Palmer was deeply interested in several metaphysical healing practices including magnetic healing, phrenology (diagnosis by reading the bumps on one's head) and spiritualism.

By 1896, a small school was opened by D. D. Palmer to teach his method. Ten years later, he was jailed for practicing medicine without a license.

The first chiropractors claimed they could cure every disease, because they thought all maladies stemmed from what they called the "subluxation of the spinal bones." Today, scientifically oriented chiropractors see their treatments as relieving muscle spasms and nerve irritation. But the problem is getting chiropractors to confine their therapy to the musculo-skeletal system where their treatments and training are proven to be effective.

According to the *Encyclopedia of Alternative Health Care*, chiropractic is the Western world's third largest primary health care profession, right after medicine and dentistry. Chiropractors are famous for skeletal manipulation, their main method being the adjustment of the spinal column to mend abnormal functioning of the nervous system.

Chiropractors are quick to point out that what they provide is a non-invasive approach to restoring and maintaining good health. It is, they say, a natural health care method which excludes drugs and surgery—although many do deal heavily in herbs and vitamin preparations which they sell out of their office. Chiropractors believe they look holistically at their patients, that they consider all aspects of their patients' lives from work to life-style to diet to exercise to emotional stress.

According to them, everyone, it seems, needs to be treated by a chiropractor. "The following three criteria are used by chiropractors when determining whether a patient is or is not a chiropractic case: (1) determine if the person has a spinal column; (2) determine if the patient has a nervous system; (3) determine if the patient is living."[4]

Little wonder some chiropractors have gotten into trouble by referring to themselves as "family physicians." Certainly they are trained: six years of college study including internships, followed by additional training for some. Chiropractors are licensed and regulated by state chiropractor boards, and they treat a wide range of patients. However, to claim that they are qualified to diagnose and treat the majority of health problems is indeed a far-fetched statement.

Interestingly, many chiropractors hardly consider diagnosis necessary at all. They still cling to D. D. Palmer's theory that virtually all disease is caused by pressure on the spinal nerves by off-centered vertebrae. No need to focus on a patient's symptoms. The cure for everything is the same—align the spine.

Chiropractic treatments run the gamut from the accepted to the absurd. Often the treatment works, whatever it may be. No wonder. The natural course of most common back problems, for instance, has been well described in medical literature. Three quarters of patients with low-back pain return to work within a month. By the end of two months, it's more than 90 percent. Only a handful continue to suffer pain. What chiropractic therapy does in many cases is parallel the course of untreated back pain. A chiropractor sees a patient three times a week for a month, twice a week for another month, then once a week for the third month. When the patient's pain eases, then ends, he naturally assumes it was the treatment that helped instead of nature running its course.

Unfortunately, some chiropractors—like Dottie's—don't stop treatments when the pain is gone. Others treat non-existent problems. Others—like Steve's—treat problems totally out of their realm of expertise.

Is Chiropractic Medically Sound?

In 1963, in direct response to chiropractic's growing popularity, an American Medical Association committee on quackery was founded. The association labeled chiropractic "an unscientific cult," and at one time barred its members from associating with or referring clients to a chiropractor. But just eleven years later, undoubtedly because of the chiropractors' strong lobbying efforts, Congress voted to allow chiropractic treatment to be covered by Medicare. With this type of precedent, what will we be paying for a decade from now?

A series of state and federal lawsuits were filed alleging that the AMA, the American Hospital Association, and various other medical associations had violated the anti-trust laws. The AMA eventually bowed to the pressure and agreed to allow its members to associate with any legally sanctioned health care professional, including chiropractors. They also agreed officially to stop calling chiropractors "unscientific." Quite a testimonial to the powerful lobbying abilities of the chiropractic movement.

Certainly chiropractors can provide help for some people with musculo-skeletal sprains and strains. The problem is that there is a tendency among chiropractors to get involved in cult nutrition, and to use excess vitamins, herbs, and other highly questionable nutritional supplements.

A certain group of chiropractors shows a definite willingness to embrace the methods of the New Age health movement— kinesiology, therapeutic touch, touch for health, naturopathic methods, and the underlying aspect of the manipulation of energy. Certainly the New Age health movement has reached out to chiropractors with open arms. And for good reason. New Age influenced chiropractors lend credibility to the New Age health movement.

A major complaint about chiropractors is their tendency to overuse large x-rays, called "spine-o-graphs," of the entire spinal column. A concerned chiropractor, Mark Sanders, D.C., wrote that these high dose radiation x-rays are often used to evaluate localized problems such as neck pain. He also states that increased x-ray usage is frequently recommended by chiropractic "practice builders" to increase revenue.

It is amazing that many people who publicly demonstrate against nuclear energy plants willingly submit to harmful irradiation by chiropractors. It is startling that parents allow their innocent children to receive such irradiation. No doubt it was never explained to these people that the radiation from a full spine x-ray is 10 to 1,000 times as much radiation as a routine chest x-ray.[5]

Another problem is the emphasis that chiropractic officials, educators, and practitioners increasingly place on casting chiropractors in the roll of primary physician rather than a muscle and joint practitioner. They emphasize that chiropractors serve as one of the "portals of entry" into the health care system, and actually function as family doctors in many cases. What they don't mention is that chiropractors have much less training in diagnosis and treatment than do physicians, that they are in no way fully licensed to practice medicine, and that they certainly are not family physicians.

At the end of the 19th century, as the scientific revolution extended the boundaries of medicine, osteopathic medicine was able to adapt to the change by incorporating scientific medicine within its realm of manipulative healing. Chiropractic, however, chose not to make that transition.

"But If He's a Christian . . ."

Texe Marrs, author of a number of books on the New Age movement, received a letter from a couple who had read some of his writings. They expressed respectful concern about some of his statements about chiropractors. "Our chiropractor is a devout Baptist who loves the Lord Jesus with all his heart," they wrote. "We share precious experiences with him and his wife. Another chiropractor friend is also a Christian. We share Christian music together. He's had a very difficult time in life and has learned to depend totally on Jesus for sustenance."

This couple makes a valid point. When it comes to alternative medicine and alternative practitioners, it's unfair to speak in generalities.

The letter goes on to say, "I know many doctors who are not involved in the New Age. I don't know any who are, though I am sure that they, as with anyone else, are subject to the deception."

Despite this testimonial, the facts are that New Age healing methods and aspects of occult spirituality are widespread throughout the chiropractic profession. Consider this statement made by a member of the Michigan Board of Chiropractic Examiners and published in the *American Chiropractic Association's Journal* in 1989:

When a vertebral adjustment is given to the patient, you are releasing the Infinite Wisdom of the Universe within that individual and the universe. Once his chronic subluxation is corrected, man will think healthy thoughts and the world will then be brought into a state of harmony. Not only will living man be healthy, but society at large will express harmony and peace.[6]

A policy statement issued by the Christian Chiropractic Association (CCA) makes it clear they are acutely aware of the New Age inroads into their profession. It has adopted guidelines in identifying New Age healing, denouncing healing that applies occult principles or energy fields or reincarnation, healing which depends on the power of the mind, and healing which includes any anti-Christian religious beliefs.

Since there is such a wide variation of practitioners gathered under the term "chiropractor," anyone considering using their services has a special responsibility to evaluate their methods as well as their orientation.

CLEANSING ENEMAS

Eugene was presented with an ultimatum: have surgery or prepare to die young. Thirty-five year old Eugene had suffered from ulcerative colitis since he was a teenager. For several years his doctors had been trying to persuade him to have a colostomy, but he refused to consider it.

"I didn't want anything to do with the embarrassment of wearing a bag on my abdomen!" he said. Now he was forced to reconsider. At the suggestion of his wife, Eugene agreed to look into an alternative clinic.

"The man who met me there introduced himself as a doctor, though I didn't recognize the initials behind his name. We talked about my condition, and he quickly assured me he could cure me without surgery."

Just what they *would* do was less clear. The more Eugene tried to pin the man down, the more evasive he became. On one point, however, the doctor was perfectly clear. He wanted $8,000 for the treatment, and he wanted it paid in advance.

"He tried hard to pressure me into signing a contract agreeing to pay the money. I asked him if I could change my mind after thinking it over, and he said, 'Absolutely not! This is a legally binding contract!'"

The doctor finally told Eugene what one of the suggested treatments was: coffee enemas administered by a colonic therapist. Eugene said he'd have to think about it, murmured a polite goodbye, and left without signing the contract.

"The fellow was indignant," Eugene remembers. "He said I was a fool! He could cure me. What could I possibly have to think about?"

Walking out likely saved his life, Eugene was later told by a medical doctor. His colon was in such bad shape it may well have burst under the pressure of the treatment suggested.

What's the Purpose?

Coffee enemas are just one type of treatment provided by colonic therapists. The point of colonic therapy is to irrigate the patient's large intestine in an effort to wash out or detoxify it of stagnated fecal material. The goal is a full intestinal washing. Colonic therapists promote the use of regular enemas to cleanse the colon and promote health. Sometimes the therapy is touted as a cure.

The theory is this: As the body's major eliminative organ, the colon collects wastes and toxins. In time, the body is threatened with overwhelming toxemia. The absorption of the toxins can affect the immune system and contribute to ill health.

Colonic therapy must be one of the most difficult sell jobs in all the alternative health care movement. Yet it is a widely used practice. An article in the *Arizona Light* magazine, July 1989, gives hints on what to look for in a good colonic therapist. Among other things, it suggests watching for "sterile disposables, filtered water, and a clean bathroom." If it were not so pathetic, it would be downright laughable.

Colonic therapy presents us with many potential problems. A main one is the possible misdiagnosis of colon ailments, which lead to a delay in proper treatment. In the case of colon cancer, this would almost certainly be fatal. Another difficulty is the possible existence of some inflammatory bowel disease, such as Crohn's disease or ulcerative colitis (which was Eugene's condition). Add to these the fact that the treatment itself is a miserable one. Why, we must wonder, would anyone ever undergo such a procedure?

HERBALISM

Today's herbalism often consists of questionable information, folklore, superstition, wishful thinking, and perhaps even outright fakery. The term *herbalism* now refers to crude drugs of vegetable origin, selected and used to treat disease—often those of a chronic nature—or to attain or maintain good health.

Worldwide it has been estimated that 75 to 80 percent of the world's population uses some form of herbal medicine. It's no wonder. In many developing countries, herbal remedies are all that's available, and they are far less expensive than drugs produced in more advanced nations. What is surprising is that with scientifically produced and tested drugs readily available, Americans are turning back to herbal treatments.

Kevin Baadsgaard, director of marketing for Nature's Sunshine Products, the largest encapsulator of dehydrated herbs in the country, says that orthodox, mainstream medicine has become so expensive that people are looking for an alternative. He goes on to say that the natural food industry is growing at a rate of about 15 to 20 percent a year. Whatever the reason for this, it is clearly big business.[7]

Unfortunately, a number of serious problems have been attributed to the inappropriate use of natural therapies. A case report in the *Guide to The New Medicine* tells of a forty-six-year-old woman who was diagnosed with colitis and gallbladder disease. In an effort to heal herself "naturally," she began a program of eating fresh fruits and drinking juices, supplemented with nutritional preparations. Then her practitioner advised her to start regular coffee enemas, which she did to the tune of ten to twelve treatments on the first night. Her body became so depleted of essential electrolytes that she suffered a seizure. She was rushed to the hospital in a coma, but despite heroic efforts to restore her internal electrolyte balance, she died.

Many people assume that "all natural" means healthy, or at least safe. This can be a tragic assumption. Just because something is natural doesn't mean it can be safely eaten or drunk. To make matters worse, the agencies charged with protecting our health have very little control over herbal products—not their collection, their packaging, nor their sale. We would be up in arms if there were the same level of contamination in a jar of peanut butter or a can of peas as there is in many natural products. The difference is, in many natural products, we have no way of knowing.

Plant Treatments

The holistic health movement has sparked this new interest in natural medicines. Holistic practitioners frequently use herbs and plants to cure. Most homeopathic remedies are plant based, and naturopathy incorporates plants into its nature cures. Iridologists, frequently claiming also to be nutritionists and herbalists, recommend plant remedies they say are required by what they find in the eyes. Aroma therapists typically prescribe inhaling the steam from heated oils and various plants—flower remedies are the homeopathic version of herbalism.

Herbalists are steeped in tradition: Chinese herbalists use carefully formulated combinations, whereas English herbalists tend to use a single herb for a specific ailment. Ayurvedic medical practitioners combine herbal remedies with purification rituals, even prescribing herbal sweat baths to rid the patient of "toxins." The herbs are available in a variety of forms: ointments and salves, plants brewed into tea, barks and roots and leaves to be chewed or inhaled, steamed herbs, capsules and tablets, douches, enemas, rectal and vaginal suppositories, herbal baths, even poultices.

The very fact that herbs are selected and prepared by lay persons presents a danger. The problem is heightened by the misleading statements made in modern herbal literature which can cause harm to those who use the herbs. For example, one article stated that diabetes is caused by parasites invading the pancreas, and that these can be driven out by pumpkin seeds or black walnuts.

In *Potter's New Encyclopedia of Botanical Drugs and Preparations,* the Wrens state that the "burdock root will wonderfully help the bites of snakes and mad dogs." In *Herbs, Medicine and Mysticism,* Leeks advises that "poke root is a valuable remedy for scabies, ulcers, ringworm, rheumatism, dysmenorrhea, and dyspepsia." While you're playing around with these things instead of getting appropriate medical care, someone could die.

Some herbs cause allergies. Others produce hormone-like effects. Still others can cause birth defects when used by pregnant women. A number of herbal preparations are actually carcinogenic. How pitiful that so many well-intentioned people turn to herbal remedies because they are convinced that, since herbs are natural, they must be safe.

The National Council Against Health Fraud consumer protection law holds that practicing medicine is a privilege, not a right, and that the state has a compelling responsibility to protect vulnerable people and their children from the glib purveyors of pseudo-medicine. But where is the regulation of practitioners such as the herbalists? No doubt many of them truly believe what they practice and preach. So what? It matters not that they are sincere in their beliefs. In fact, the true believers may well be the most deadly of all. Zealotry can be more dangerous than fraud.

HOMEOPATHY

"I have gone to countless doctors and each one gave me tranquilizers, antidepressants, and stuff," a young woman wrote in a letter to me. "I was very dissatisfied with taking drugs and having their side effects. So, for the last five years I have been going to a homeopathic doctor and using remedies that are supposed to be more natural with no bad side effects. When I go to the homeopath, he asks me questions about how I feel, what I eat, etc. Then he tests me on a machine that uses my energy, and it tells him what area my body is weak in. It might be my liver, for example, or my stomach.

"I read a book on New Age Medicine, and homeopathy was lightly touched on. Now I'm asking you, is homeopathic a form of witchcraft? Am I dabbling in something, unaware that I'm going against God's Word? I'm torn about what to do because I have believed in homeopathic for over five years and have been pretty much brainwashed that homeopathic is okay because it is a natural healer. But somehow I am disturbed by it, and am wondering if there is more to it than I know.

"Interestingly enough, my homeopathic doctor claims to be a Christian. I even saw his staff gathered in prayer before the work day started. I guess this concerned me. Is it all okay?"

This young lady brings up some interesting questions. Just what is homeopathy? Is it Christian? Is it scientific? Can a patient be a Christian and still be involved in homeopathic therapy?

Red Flags from the Beginning

Homeopathic medicine is an example of an early alternative split from conventional medicine. In homeopathy we see many of the typical holistic characteristics such as the "eureka discovery," deduction of theory from therapy, worship of the "natural," documentation by anecdote, and reliance on spiritual and energy forces for healing.

Like naturopathic medicine, homeopathic medicine arose in

the age of so-called heroic medicine. It was an outgrowth of a movement against medical practices of that day, with all of its harmful side effects of bleeding and cupping (to get rid of "bad blood" that caused disease), purgatives and laxatives, and numerous other extreme medical interventions.

It all began in the late 1700s with the concepts of Samuel Hahnemann, a German physician who saw illness as an expression of disorder within the "vital force" of the body. He considered symptoms of disease to be positive expressions of the body's own healing capacity. While traditional medicine studied individuals with diseases, Hahnemann studied normal people. He came up with some rather startling conclusions.

Hahnemann was a deeply religious man, steeped in the mysticism of Emmanuel Swedenborg, an eighteenth century scientist, philosopher, and mystic. Hahnemann believed healing came from God and nature, and needed only to be gently encouraged by the physician.

Laws of Homeopathy

A basic concept of homeopathy for which Hahnemann has become known is what he called "the law of similars." That is, diseases are cured by agents capable of symptoms resembling those found in the disease under treatment. Upon this basis, he founded and coined the new word "homeopathy" to describe medical treatment based on the law of similars.

As Hahnemann began to practice this on his patients, he came to believe that by reducing the dosages of his remedies, they would become even more powerful. He also began to believe that spiritual reality was more important than material reality. Therefore, he came to regard the "spiritual essence" of a drug as more important than its physical substance.

This phenomenon led Hahnemann to the second law of homeopathy, known as "the law of infinitesimals." This law states that the smaller the dose of a remedy, when properly diluted, the more effective it will be at stimulating the body's vital forces to react against disease.

Hahnemann insisted that not only the diluted medicine but the actual process of diluting a medicine—the shaking and mixing—imparted healing power to the substance. According to the law of infinitesimals, each succeeding dilution will be more powerful than the last. He also proposed a rule for treatment with these diluted drugs: "the single remedy rule," he called it. The homeopathic physician, he said, should use only one remedy at a time, waiting to see what happens before taking further actions.

There were other laws, too, including "the law of chronic disease." This law states that when disease persists despite treatment, it is the result of one or more conditions that affect many people, and that these conditions have been driven deep inside the body by earlier medical therapy. What an incredible out! Whenever Hahnemann's methods failed, he simply blamed it on the patient's previous treatment.

The British Royal family is still treated by a homeopathic physician. Queen Elizabeth II is said always to travel with a homeopathic first aid kit. In America, homeopathy is again on the rise. Here practitioners are primarily non-M.D.s, including naturopaths and chiropractors.

The theories of homeopathy present us with many problems. First, they don't stand up to scientific evaluation. Using the law of infinitesimal, natural substances are diluted over and over until at the twenty-fourth time, it is so diluted that it is possible that not even a single molecule of the original substance is to be found in the alcohol or water mixture. No matter. Homeopathic practitioners claim that the more it is diluted, the deeper acting the remedy. (Find this hard to understand? That should signal a red flag.)

The Answer to Disease?

Homeopathy has a third great doctrine, one that homeopaths don't talk much about. Yet it was this doctrine upon which Hahnemann hung his hat. He said, "Seven eighths of all chronic diseases are produced by the existence in the system of that infectious disorder known in the language of science by the appelation of Psora."[8] According to Hahnemann's writings, "psora" was the fundamental cause of countless other diseases, including insanity, depression, cancer, gout, asthma, paralysis, and pains of every kind. In other words, Hahnemann claimed to have found the ultimate answer to disease itself.

This idea of one overall cause of disease and therefore a single cure is ludicrous. In light of medical science, most of Hahnemann's principles would meet with similar skepticism were they as widely promoted as the homeopathic remedies themselves.

Homeopathic principles state that the medicine and the dose used to treat a disease must be highly individualized for each patient. This is to be determined through painstaking examination by a doctor specially trained in homeopathy. Yet many homeopathic drugs are now being marketed over the counter, even for such serious conditions as cancer and heart and kidney disease. Health food stores across the nation sell such potions as extract of tarantula—a supposed treatment for multiple sclerosis, and extract of cobra venom—touted as a cancer treatment. Home remedy kits and books abound, including one which suggests that stroke victims take one homeopathic remedy to allay anxiety and another to encourage healing of a brain injury. So much for individualized medicine!

Homeopathic practitioners have a great deal of derision for traditional physicians who treat patients with multiple medications. It is the stimulation of the person's immune system by the homeopathic medicines, they claim, that make their diluted portions work. Never mind that it's all a totally unproven theory, and that the medicine they offer is little more than high-priced water.

"At Least It's Safe"

A young woman wrote to us stating she was attracted to homeopathic medicine because she considered it entirely safe. Of course, it is safe! Since when is drinking water dangerous? But *is* homeopathy safe? Are you willing to forego real medicine and a real cure? Are you willing to bet your life on it?

Homeopathic philosophy is straight out of energy therapies. These concepts are based on monism, the belief that everything in the universe, including God, is one and the same. The Chinese call it Chi, the Japanese call it Kai, and it's the prana of Ayurvedic medicine.

How it's all supposed to work isn't explained to patients who use homeopathy. All they're told is that it works. In fact, homeopathic practitioners like to say that most pharmacologists don't understand how and why most drugs work, either. Well, this may be true of the individual pharmacist in your corner drugstore, but for most medication today, there is much more than a mere theory as to why it works.

When he was challenged about the exceedingly diluted doses he used, Hahnemann insisted that the curative powers of the drug lay not in the presence of the original active ingredient, but in the physician's method of preparing the dose. A simple dilution just wasn't sufficient. The vial containing the medicine had to be struck against a leather pad a number of times so that the drug could be "dynamized" and act "spiritually upon the vital forces" of the body.

Today, when homeopaths are asked the same question, they explain that something remains. The "essence" of the substance is still there—its energy, or its pattern.

Both Hahnemann's assertion and the more modern homeopathic explanation take us directly into the realm of the supernatural. No natural power could allow for a substance not present in a solution to continue to exert its effect, nor could it act spiritually upon the body's vital forces.

Andrew Weil, M.D., is one who claims to understand homeopathic therapy. He practices it and he teaches it. He writes:

> Homeopaths use remedies containing no drug materials, yet they believe in the existence and therapeutic power of some other aspect of the drug—of its idea, if you will, or its ghost or spirit.

Truly, homeopathy is spiritual medicine consistent with its founder's views on the relative importance of spiritual verses material reality.[9]

Spiritual? Absolutely! Christian? Definitely not! Its spirituality is not at all as that defined by the Bible, but as defined by Samuel Hahnemann and his modern day homeopaths.

MACROBIOTICS

Bonlyn Walls knows about macrobiotics. After a painful divorce, she was searching for a church home. Raised in a Presbyterian family and married in a Catholic church, she says she "walked the aisle" in high school. It never really changed her life.

Bonlyn found her local New Age food store with its variety of new foods extremely tempting. She found it spiritually attractive as well. Many of her friends attended a Unity church, and some were engaged in open marriage situations. She herself had consulted a channeler, and became involved in the Unity church.

"There were lots of reasons I started the macrobiotic diet," Bonlyn said. "For one thing, I was looking for a low-sugar diet. And I liked vegetables and fruits and whole grain foods." Certainly nothing is wrong with this. Those are the same reasons our family occasionally shops at the whole foods store here in Austin.

As a teacher in public school, Bonlyn met two very caring compassionate teachers who shared a lot of New Age ideas with her. One was involved in macrobiotics. Bonlyn asked questions about this new method of cooking and eating.

She was attracted to it partly because her new husband needed to lose weight and wasn't feeling very well. Anyway, she had been raised to avoid junk food. Before long she became wholeheartedly involved in macrobiotics.

"I tried so hard to be perfect at everything I did," Bonlyn told me. "I was really attracted to a diet such as this that claims to be better, safer, cleaner, and helpful to the earth, too." She had no idea there were any religious connotations in the yin and yang principles of preparing food macrobiotically.

A Diet, a Philosophy

At first, in the excitement of the new foods and the unique ways of preparing them, Bonlyn glossed over the references to yin/yang balance, the healing properties of certain foods, the emphasis on concepts that had to do with the healing of the earth, and certainly any religious concepts. But one day, while leafing through a new cookbook, she was amazed to find references to reincarnation.

"I spent an awful lot of time on my diet," she told me. "Looking back, that diet became an idol to me. I ate macrobiotically to save myself from disease and an uncaring environment, to avoid modern fast-paced consciousness, and from a deeply spiritual connection to the earth, to my food, and to my own existence."

It was as Bonlyn listened on the radio to a talk about the New Age Movement and about a book by Texe Marrs, *Dark Secrets of the New Age,* that she suddenly grew alarmed. "I read the book cover to cover," she said. "Then I discussed it with a friend, then with a Christian pastor, then with my counselor."

For years Bonlyn had been seeing Ted and Nancy, professional counselors. Together they read *Unlimited Power,* a book by Anthony Robbins, a nationally known motivational speaker whose techniques include walking across hot coals barefooted to increase personal esteem.

"I did have some misgivings about the group," she admits. "I wasn't too sure about the book, either. Nancy had attended training on neurolinguistics, and she incorporated its practices into our group. I was really amazed at how involved she and Ted were becoming."

Even though she was uneasy, Bonlyn wanted to stay in the group. "I really needed to work on my relationship with my mother."

Still, she was having more and more doubts.

Bonlyn called up a friend, and through a series of remarkable "coincidences," she started attending a Bible study with her. The topic under discussion was a relevant one—spiritual warfare.

"The more we got into the Bible, the more uncomfortable I got in those counseling sessions," Bonlyn told me.

She wrote a letter to her counselor, Ted, and told him she was sorry for having given him a diet book that mentioned reincarnation. When she met with Ted, Bonlyn asked if he had gotten her letter about the book. He had, but he said he hadn't read the book. At any rate, he didn't have any trouble with the New Age thought, he told her.

More and more disturbed and uncomfortable, Bonlyn decided to drop out of the counseling group. "I went to Ted and thanked him for all the times he had helped me. I couldn't believe it when he said he was sick of my religiosity, then added that he was really hurt and distressed."

Instead of going back to Ted or Nancy, Bonlyn went to see a Christian counselor. Finally there was someone who understood what was happening to her. Finally she got some help.

Today Bonlyn says, "Without the Lord Jesus in my life I would be fair game for any satanic device."

Bonlyn's transition out of the macrobiotic diet life-style was a quick one. She started by getting rid of all her cookbooks. She eats healthfully, but isn't compulsive about it.

Bonlyn doesn't blame Ted and Nancy for all her problems. She doesn't even blame the macrobiotic diet. "But," she says, "that diet was a very real snare to me."

The Macrobiotic "Cure"

Macrobiotic therapy is probably the most common dietary cancer remedy in the United States today. Not only is it purported to prevent cancer, it's touted as a cancer cure. "If diet causes cancer," many people simplistically reason, "then it must be able to cure cancer."

Proponents claim that food intake must be carefully balanced to counteract disease. The following ad ran in *East-West* magazine, a large circulation New Age publication: "Food is medicine. Today modern science and medicine have begun to agree with this ancient wisdom. More and more people are realizing that diet is directly connected with our health and well-being. What we eat, what's in it and how it's made is so very important. This is the macrobiotic point of view."

This may indeed be the macrobiotic point of view. But for the all encompassing life-style known as macrobiotics, it is only the beginning. And it is definitely not endorsed by modern science and medicine.

The notion of balance is central to macrobiotic treatment. Yin foods are prescribed for yang cancers, and yang foods are prescribed for yin cancers.

A patient who strictly adhered to the macrobiotic diet actually died of malnutrition. Subsequently the diet was expanded to include a few more foods. Yet nutritional deficiency is still a potential result of this dietary "cure." It is especially hazardous for either surgical or cancer patients who already have an increased need for nutrients.

Who Made the Diagnosis?

When we hear the glowing reports of cancer cured by a macrobiotic diet, we must ask: Who diagnosed that cancer? Often it's the macrobiotic practitioners themselves, and they frequently use methods that are both unscientific and unproven. Some are downright false. Obviously their stories of "cures" are likely as questionable as their diagnostic methods.

The American Cancer Society has found absolutely no evidence that the macrobiotic diet can benefit a person suffering from cancer. In fact, they go a step further by strongly urging individuals with cancer not to participate in treatments with macrobiotic diets. In 1988, the U.S. General Surgeon said, "There is no credible evidence that nutritional changes specifically help in the cure of cancer patients."[10]

So Just What Is Macrobiotics?

Briefly put, it's an idiosyncratic version of the ancient concept of yin and yang. According to oriental philosophy, yin and yang are opposing yet complimentary forces which are presumed to exist throughout all elements of the universe. It's necessary to maintain a balance and harmony between yin and yang, they say, in order to adapt to one's environment. In this philosophy, many things are grouped according to yin and yang—diseases, bodily organs, food items, food color, form and shape, growing seasons. Everything is assigned yin and yang qualities.

In dietary counseling and practice, these designations are used to explain how a supposed imbalance in the diet results in a health disorder. The imbalance isn't explained nutritionally, understand. It is explained philosophically.

Here's where the diagnosis comes in. Macrobiotic diagnosis is essential if the correct diet is to be prescribed. The counselors use such unscientific methods as iridology and the reading of the face to determine internal problems. For example, a swelling or discoloration on the upper bridge of the nose and the outside of the temples, blisters on the eyes or a blue-grey color in the middle regions of the white of the eye, brings a diagnosis of pancreatic cancer.

Needless to say, such techniques are highly suspect. The practice of iridology has been proven time and time again to be totally inaccurate in diagnosing illness. And yet, through such measures, many ailments are "diagnosed," and of course "appropriate" dietary treatment is prescribed by macrobiotic practitioners.

And Those Who Fail?

Can you guess which patients are considered "macrobiotically terminal"? The ones who make mistakes in preparing their food or those who stray from the diet or those who lack the support of their families—especially family members who prepare the macrobiotic food. In fact, family members who don't go on the macrobiotic diet are encouraged to move out until the patient has recovered. It just may be their fault that healing hasn't come. Sound familiar? That's New Age rhetoric: shift the blame for failure to something other than the treatment.

If it's not the fault of family members, then it must be the fault of the patient. Mishio Kushi, a leading proponent of macrobiotic in America, advised his patients, "Admit that the food that has been consumed and the previous life-style are what led to his or her present condition."[11]

According to one of Kushi's seminars, "The secret to turn sickness to health, suffering to happiness, poverty to prosperity, and war to peace, all depends on the understanding and practice of this infinite order." And how do we tap into this secret? It's easy, says Kushi. "We lead our life in a simple modest way, eating macrobiotically and develop a spirit of gratitude to everyone and everything. This way, it becomes easy to attain the order of the infinite universe which is our life itself—eternal and everlasting."[12]

Macrobiotics just a diet? Don't you believe it! For Kushi and many others, macrobiotics is a spiritual commitment through which they seek a unification of thought and purpose in what they call a "new planetary civilization." Kushi entices those interested in macrobiotics by saying, "Until now, I have taught only about 20 percent of what I wish to leave behind. . . . Let's study together the laws and principles of the invisible world in preparation for the next stage in our endless journey through the stars."[13]

NATUROPATHY

Naturopathy, a term coined by a nineteenth century German, was first taught in America by Benedict Lust. He founded the American School of Naturopathy in New York City in 1902. Today, naturopathic medicine is considered legal in six states and the District of Columbia. Many naturopaths practice in other states under the original "drugless therapy" license issued before laws prohibiting naturopathic practices went into effect.

Typically, naturopaths use standard laboratory tests and clinical examinations to determine the course of treatment. They also use such "diagnostic" methods as iridology, an examination of the iris of the eye, to tell where in the body there is a problem. One must question a practitioner's ability to interpret even standard laboratory data when he would use so blatantly an unscientific method such as iridology. It should also send a red flag flying high.

Three Basic Principles

The driving principle behind naturopathy is the healing power of nature. Its three basic principles are: (1) The body has a natural drive to maintain equilibrium—symptoms of disease are only indications that the body is striving to heal itself. (2) The root of all disease is the accumulation of waste products and toxins due to poor life-style habits. (3) The body contains both the wisdom and the power to heal itself—provided one does what enhances rather than what interferes with this power.

A naturopath believes in a world of physical toxins in which most people are poisoning themselves through what they eat. Foods filled with additives, high in sugar, and low in fiber are the culprits, they say.

Now, as a physician, I'm certainly interested in seeing a person achieve a low fat, high fiber diet. There are well documented reasons for this. Studies show we can reduce our risk of cancer of the colon with such a diet. It has been proven that a low fat diet can reduce your risk of heart disease. What is not proven is the importance naturopaths place on various toxins, both those which occur naturally within the body and those that come from such external sources as pesticides and chemicals.

Naturopathic Training

What are naturopaths trained to do? Well, they take such courses as gastroenterology, cardiology, minor surgery, clinical nutrition. All pretty typically mainstream sounding, isn't it? It seems to fit right in with modern medical theory. However, they also study a core of natural therapeutics ranging from homeopathy to Chinese medicine, hydrotherapy, and manipulative therapy. Many are involved in reflexology, acupressure, acupuncture, biofeedback, meditation, yoga exercises, physiotherapy, and especially herbal therapy. These practices are definitely not mainstream. (We recently had a phone conversation with a local naturopath who had a doctor of divinity degree and who claimed he could heal AIDS over the telephone. It's reassuring to the ill in our community that help is only a phone call away.)

Naturopathy, in a throwback to nineteenth century medicine, believes that fasting and purging are necessary to rid the body of previous poisons. Naturopaths in America today not only believe in nature cure—a natural diet, fresh air, exercise, and relaxation. (Not many problems yet.) They also add certain "remedial measures" such as herbal treatments, chiropractic manipulation, and acupuncture.

Now that Laetrile has fallen upon poor press, and Americans are finally realizing that there was no miracle in this so-called miracle cure for cancer, a new approach is making its appearance. A June 17, 1982, article in *The New England Journal of Medicine* discusses this "natural" approach to malignant disease that emphasizes cure through purification and the body's capacity to heal itself. The article noted that these remedies are rooted in homeopathic and naturopathic beliefs, Indian and oriental philosophy, and nineteenth century theories of intestinal putrification, and that the Federal Drug Administration and federal government are looking into the regimens suggested.

What are these regimens of natural healing? They are purification through diet, detoxification and internal cleansing, and mind control.

Naturopaths would like to cast themselves more and more in the roll of primary physicians. In the October 11, 1976, issue of *U.S. News and World Report,* a recent president of the national organization of naturopaths was quoted as saying, "Naturopaths can and do diagnose. They apply naturopathic therapy, too, and thereby treat acute infectious disease and abnormalities of the digestive system, the respiratory system, the cardiovascular system, the urinary system, the hemopoietic system, the nervous system, and the endocrine system."

The Immunization Problem

Many naturopaths are reluctant to support vaccination treatments, even for the routine prevention of such things as measles, mumps, polio, tetanus, diptheria and pertussus. In fact, some naturopaths view vaccines as being "essentially a pinnacle type hierarchical system with a very clear, authority figure and people subservient to the authority. Injections are only available on a prescription basis."[14]

The increasing acceptance of naturopaths in this nation, with their negative stand on vaccines, poses an increasing danger to the children of today's society—and so to society as a whole. We are no longer petrified by the sheet horror of these "routinely" immunizable diseases because over the last half century we have basically wiped them out of developed countries. The little girl down the street isn't crippled by polio. The neighbors aren't quarantined for diptheria. These killers of the past have lost their sting—at least temporarily. Why? Because of rigorous immunization programs. To discontinue these programs would be more than senseless; it would be downright criminal.

NATURE'S WAY

Healing nature's way? It does sound good. And it's true that some old home remedies really do help. A bowl of hot chicken soup will do as much good for a cold as anything else. Yet many natural preparations will do little for the patient. Others can make the patient worse. Some can kill.

The fact is, nature is "fallen," according to the Bible. Expelled from Paradise, man has had to learn to wrest from nature good farming land, tolerable living conditions—and disease-fighting drugs. A gracious God has given us both the raw material and the ability to develop such technologies as medical science. Why deny ourselves such gifts, in a misguided attempt to return to a naive concept of nature?

Chapter Six

CAN YOU THINK YOURSELF WELL?

Mind Therapies

"**M**atthew, you can't be sick. God didn't make disease, and you live in the kingdom of God."

As the Christian Science practitioner treated tiny Matthew Swan, the fifteen-month-old child lay still on a couch, his clothes soaked with perspiration from his soaring fever.

Other practitioners had treated the baby before, and his fever had always gone down. Now, for the fourth time in a matter of months, a Christian Science practitioner was working to change the tiny child's mind so that he wouldn't believe in disease.

"I'm afraid Christian Science isn't working. It's not healing Matthew," the boy's mother confessed to the practitioner. She had been raised to believe, not to question.

The practitioner was certain she knew the root of Matthew's problem: his mother and father. Their fears and doubts were causing the boy's symptoms and interfering with his treatment, the practitioner maintained.

"All false, negative beliefs have to be discarded," she told them sternly. "Think positively and don't complain."

Matthew's mother couldn't help fearing for her son. "But I

was even more afraid of the doctor, and what would happen if I didn't trust fully," she now admits. The Christian Science church teaches that God and doctors are mutually exclusive. "If we went to a doctor, our church would desert us," Mrs. Swan said.

Meanwhile, Matthew continued to get worse and worse. On the sixth day, the early morning silence was pierced by his shrill screams of pain. His terrified parents called a Christian Science nurse. She was soothing and comforting, and assured them they were doing everything right.

The following day the practitioner came by again. "I have healed your son," she announced confidently.

His parents weren't so sure. Now totally incoherent, Matthew was thrashing about wildly in his crib.

When Matthew's distraught parents finally took their son to a real doctor, everyone in the clinic was shocked at the baby's condition. "It's meningitis," the doctor said. The team got permission from the Swans to perform emergency neurosurgery on their son immediately, to drain the abscesses in his brain. Among themselves, the medical personnel whispered that it was probably already too late.

Five days later, nearly three weeks after his fever first struck, Matthew Swan died.[1]

POWERS OF THE MIND

"Experience hundreds of modern health miracles!" proclaims the ad for the medical self-help book *Positive Living and Health,* from the editors of *Prevention* magazine. "Halt a headache with the touch of your hand. Use willpower alone to lower blood pressure or cholesterol. Program your own mind to reverse powerful ills, like cancer." This is only the beginning. You name the ailment, this book tells you how to cure it.

A recently published ad encourages readers to discover the story of a young blind woman who learned to drive just with the power of her mind. And that's only the beginning. It also promises "Thousands of instant miracle mind cures. Instantly have a super memory. Instantly lose weight naturally. Instantly relieve stress and boost your brain power. Just sit back, close your eyes and soak in the secrets."

Newspaper headlines extol the message. It comes over our televisions, in our newspapers and magazines: Our minds can heal us.

Recently a number of books, some written by physicians, have promoted this belief that the mind can indeed heal the body. The enthralled public has responded by making several of these books best-sellers.

Power over the mind is a goal of many alternative healing techniques. But now mainstream medicine is also becoming interested in the mind/body connection. Studies have been published in the *Journal of the American Medical Association* on a combination of meditation, yoga, and a vegetarian diet to reverse blockages in the coronary arteries, even a study exploring whether the elderly can delay death until after an important event.

What is power of the mind? Is it just an elaboration on the old mind over matter maxim?

The idea that the mind and body are connected goes back thousands of years. Hypnosis, meditation, biofeedback—all these have been applied with some success to conditions many consider somewhat psychosomatic in nature. Asthmatics have found relief through relaxation exercises. Hypertensive patients have lowered their blood pressure. Migraine sufferers have controlled their headaches. The difference is that now some insist that mind power techniques are just as good for such conditions as cancer and AIDS.

Bernie Siegel, M.D., the Drs. Simonton, and AIDS counselor Louise L. Hay are just some of the professionals who are busy spreading the gospel of the healing power of the mind. All of us, they say—and this includes the terminally ill—should be able to think ourselves back to good health. All we need is the right attitude.

Mind over matter? Think yourself well? Certainly it's not all bad, but we do need to take a balanced approach. To believe all illnesses can be thought away can be a deadly oversimplification.

ANATOMY OF A DELUSION

Phineas Quimby, a mid-nineteenth-century clock maker in Belfast, Maine, was dying of tuberculosis. When he heard of a friend who had cured himself by riding a horse, Quimby decided to cure himself by riding in a horse-drawn carriage.

About two miles from the stable, the horse refused to walk up a hill. Quimby was forced to walk most of the way with the horse by his side. By the time he reached the top, Quimby was so exhausted he barely had the strength to lift the whip. After a passing farmer came by and got him started moving again, Quimby reported, "Excitement took possession of my senses and I drove the horse as fast as I could go uphill and down until I reached home. When I got into the stable, I felt as strong as ever."

This experience caused Quimby to doubt the medical profession's ability to diagnosis and effectively cure disease. From this doubt arose what he termed "The Mental Healing of Mind Cure Movement."

Quimby was convinced that disease was not caused by physical disorders at all. It was caused by false belief. If we could just eliminate the false belief, he insisted, we would eliminate the primary cause of disease.

In 1859, Quimby moved to Portland, Maine, where he began a practice based on his unique method of healing through the mind. Four of his many patients, one of which was Mary Baker Patterson, later to become Mary Baker Eddy, founder of Christian Science, became key figures in spreading his thought.

Today's advocates of thinking yourself well suggest that if all stages of disease are psychosomatic, then all causes of disease are psychosomatic. How long a person suffers with the disease is also psychosomatic, and so is the healing process. In other words, the mind completely controls the disease. To follow this line of thinking, you're sick because you think you are. Although Dr. Kenneth Pelletier, author of *Holistic Medicine,* does not deny that bacteria causes illness, he says individuals are susceptible to disease when their minds aren't suitably trained or ordered, when their lives are too full of stress. In other words, you are responsible not only for your illness, but also for how long it lasts and how severe it is. (Red Flag No. 3!)

Many other groups, organizations, and sects espouse this philosophy that the mind is paramount in the healing process. Author and editor Norman Cousins, after a demanding schedule in Leningrad and Moscow, found himself in what he called a state of "adrenal exhaustion." Later he claimed it was a precondition of his supposedly "progressive, incurable" collagen disease which turned out to be ankylosing spondylitis.

In an effort to cure himself, Cousins decided to put himself on a slow intravenous drip therapy of vitamin C. He rented films of *Candid Camera* and *The Three Stooges* and watched and laughed and watched and laughed. Through laughter, vitamin C, and rest, he determined to get better. In his book, *Anatomy of an Illness,* Cousins states that after months of slow recuperation, he was able to resume his work at *The Saturday Review*. Over the ensuing year, Cousins continued to laugh, and his mobility continued to improve.

Did the vitamin C or the laughter or the rest have anything to do with his recovery? Was it a combination of the three? Did he perhaps will himself well? We really don't know what helped him. But evidently he did get better, and he has reached some conclusions of his own.[2]

1. "The will to live is not a theoretical abstraction, but a physiologic reality with therapeutic characteristics." Cousins says you can actually change the physiology of your body. A thought can change the rate at which your heart beats. It can change your pulse or your immune system or your white blood count. What he doesn't mention is just how you can be certain the change is for your good.

2. "My doctor knew that his biggest job was to encourage

the patient's will to live and to mobilize all the natural resources of the body and mind to combat disease." Actually, Dr. Cousins acted as his own doctor. He's the one who prescribed the vitamin C and the movies. He placed himself at complete rest. And it was he himself who came to the conclusion that encouraging his body's natural resources was his biggest job.

3. "Since I didn't accept the verdict, I wasn't trapped in the cycle of fear, depression, and panic that frequently accompany a supposedly incurable illness." What Cousins did was to take physical action. But if all disease is psychosomatic, why did he need to take this action? Why didn't he simply will himself well? Was it because he was afraid that wouldn't be enough? Or did he have enough doubt that he decided it would be better to cover all bases?

Norman Cousins's story is a clear example of why the holistic health movement appeals to so many people. The testimonials are exciting. The anecdotes of spectacular recoveries are inspiring. People think, "If it worked for him, maybe it'll work for me. It's certainly worth a try!" Well-meaning friends and relatives bring books detailing cures attributed to vitamin C, herbal preparations, macrobiotic diets, visualization, visits to psychic healers, and so on.

What the person has really decided is that he just doesn't quite trust his physician. Not completely. He wants to be sure he's not missing out on some way to heal himself.

I can certainly understand such thoughts and feelings when a patient is faced with an apparently incurable or deadly disease. I can appreciate her panic and desperation. If she cooperated with the recommended treatment—chemotherapy, for instance—and along with that she rented some funny movies, read joke books, and took extra doses of vitamin C, what would be the harm? No harm at all. Maybe there wouldn't be any help, either, but it couldn't hurt. And all her bases would be covered.

The problem comes when alternative practices lead the patient away from scientifically proven medicine. What if, instead of just renting movies and taking vitamin C, the person decides to embark upon a course that would be harmful—financially or physically or emotionally? What if the harm would be spiritual?

Desperate people are vulnerable to spiritual and religious indoctrination. And without a doubt, religious implications abound in the field of alternative medicine. When deciding whether or not something is okay, it's not enough to simply ask, Does it work? or Will it make me worse? All the ramifications of the possible impact on the physical body, the mental self, and the spiritual soul need to be considered, both by those recommending the treatment and by those taking it.

CHRISTIAN SCIENCE

Mary Baker Eddy's loyalty to Quimby ended because of an incident that occurred less than a month after Quimby's death. In February of 1866 Mrs. Eddy fell on some ice and lost the use of her limbs. Supposedly her condition was pronounced incurable, and her physician gave her just three days to live. But, she later claimed, three days after her fall she arose from her bed completely healed. Her secret? She had read Matthew 9:2: "And behold, they brought to Him a paralytic lying on a bed. And Jesus, seeing their faith, said to the paralytic, 'Son, be of good cheer; your sins are forgiven you.'" Never mind that Eddy's attending physician later denied under oath that he ever said she was in a precarious physical position at all. In fact, he insisted, she always enjoyed robust health.

According to Mary Baker Eddy, she received a revelation when she was healed. The essence of this revelation was that the "principle or life of men is a divine intelligence and power which, understood, can heal all diseases."[3] Mrs. Eddy became a popular teacher, healer, and writer. Within a short time she disavowed Quimby altogether and claimed it was she who was the original discoverer of the science of mental healing.

Mrs. Eddy moved to Boston and founded the Church of Christ, Scientist, in 1879. In 1881 she established the Massachusetts Metaphysical College, and in 1883 *The Christian Sci-*

ence Journal was launched. It was the beginning of New Thought teaching. From it sprang such organizations as Divine Science, Unity School of Christianity, and the Church of Religious Science.

There are three major principals of New Thought teaching: (1) God is an impersonal spirit force, (2) spirit is the source and cause of the physical, and (3) thoughts have power to condition our lives.

Some groups have decided that the mind can control a lot more than just disease; it can control all aspects of living. These groups of course attribute this belief to the Creator of the Mind. Certainly Christian Science is one such group.

Mary Baker Eddy wrote: "I should blush to write of *Science and Health with Key to the Scriptures* as I have were it of human origin and I, apart from God, its author. But as I was only a scribe echoing the harmonies of heaven in divine metaphysics, I cannot be super modest of the Christian Science textbook" (*Christian Science Journal,* 1901).

What did Mrs. Eddy write under "divine inspiration"? One thing she wrote is that death is "an illusion, the life of life." Mrs. Eddy died in December of 1910.

The Christian Science Publishing Society has furnished us with a book entitled *Facts About Christian Science*. In answer to the question, What is Christian Science? they respond: "Christian Science is a religion based on the words and works of Christ Jesus. It draws its authority from the Bible, and its teachings are set forth in *Science and Health with Key to the Scriptures,* by Mary Baker Eddy." They note that "a distinctive part of Christian Science is its healing of physical disease as well as sin by spiritual means alone."

Christian Scientists believe that God created man in His own image (Gen. 1:27). Since He pronounced all He had made "very good," then man in the image of God's Spirit must be wholly spiritual and as perfect as His Creator. They believe "it follows that the sick and sinning mortal man who appears to the physical senses is a false representation of man, a material misconception of man as he really is."

The Basis of Healing

Christian Scientists do not believe their healing is based on blind faith in the unknown, but rather "on an enlightened understanding of God as infinite, divine Mind, Spirit, Soul, Principle, Life, Truth, and Love."[4] In fact, they "repudiate the use of suggestion, will power, hypnotism, and all those forms of psychotherapy which employ the human mind as a curative agent. Instead, Christian Science turns human thought to the enlightening and saving power of divine Truth." It is their belief that "sin, sickness, lack, sorrow, selfishness, ignorance, fear, and all material mindedness are included within the range of mortal errors to be corrected and overcome by scientific understanding of God."[5]

The healing aspect of their religion, say Christian Scientists, is as important as the healing ministry of Jesus in the New Testament. For them it is "the most conspicuous proof of the validity of Christian Science and is regarded as one of the natural results of drawing closer to God in one's thinking and living."[6] This is a very significant statement. It has a lot to do with the reasons why people become involved with this religion, and why they stay involved at the cost of physical pain and suffering—even death—of those around them, including their own children. Those who need help applying Christian Science to a particular problem may turn to a practitioner, one of a group of experienced Christian Scientists who devote themselves to the healing ministry, as listed in the directory of the *Christian Science Journal*. It was such a practitioner who guided the treatment of little Matthew Swan.

Can Christian Science be combined with reliance on medical aid? *Facts About Christian Science* says, "No. Christ Jesus, who never used material remedies of any sort, declared (John 6:63), 'It is the Spirit that quickeneth. The flesh profiteth nothing.' And again (Matt. 6:24), 'No man can serve two masters.'" The book goes on to say, "Experience has shown that the attempt to combine Christian Science treatment with medicine is fair to neither system and lessens the efficacy of both."[7] It is this so-called "unfair combination" that prevented baby Matthew from getting medical help.

Mrs. Eddy claimed to have restored "the power of healing to Christians." She herself professed to have healed all sorts of diseases, including cancer, tuberculosis, and diphtheria. Yet Dr. Alfred Farlow, chairman of the publications committee of the Christian Science Church and president of the mother church in Boston, testified he didn't know of a single healing of any organic disease ever having been made by Mrs. Eddy in her entire life except for a stiff leg.[8]

Even with such inconsistencies, one of the chief attractions of Christian Science is its seeming power over disease and mental conflict. Unfortunately, countless people have died because Christian Science practitioners couldn't heal their illnesses.

Who Decides for the Children?

In May, 1989, neighbors who realized they had not seen twelve-year-old Ashley King for months notified the Arizona Child Protection Services. They found the girl sick in bed. After a court ordered examination, doctors determined she had advanced bone cancer. Although she had been prayed over regularly by a Christian Science practitioner, the disease had progressed much too far to be treated. The tumor on Ashley's leg was forty-one inches in circumference. In places it had actually dissolved her bone. Even worse, the cancer had spread to her lungs. The skin on her buttocks was infected and rotting. Her heart, strained by the cancerous tumor, was failing.

"I'm in so much pain," Ashley told the doctors. "You don't know how I have suffered."

Still, instead of being hospitalized, Ashley was put into a Christian Science nursing home where the only treatment available was prayer. It's hard to imagine the agony this child endured. An entry in the nursing home log relates: "The nurse reminded the screaming child of the lateness of the hour, and that 'other patients are sleeping.'" Ashley died a few weeks later.[9]

Across the country, children lie dead because of untreated medical problems. With prompt medical treatment, many could have been cured. No one should have to suffer and die because of the religious beliefs of another.

Yet Nathan Talbott, Christian Science spokesman, says, "Children are so responsive to our methods that I think most Christian Scientists would say they are more quickly and effectively healed than adults are." Evidently he chooses to ignore the deaths of Matthew Swan, Ashley King, and many other children.

Can They Really Heal?

Christian Scientists love to quote statistics, which they believe show their healing is superior to medical care. Theirs is an interesting and selective use of statistics, for a church bylaw forbids the church to even count how many members it has. We tend to believe statistics done by objective organizations such as the *Journal of the American Medical Association*.

The journal published an article in 1989 which compared the longevity of graduates of Principia College, a Christian Science school located in Illinois, with a control group. When fifty years of alumni records were analyzed, the researcher found that both men and women graduates of Principia had significantly higher death rates than those in the non-Christian Science control group. This is particularly surprising considering the fact that most Christian Scientists neither drink nor smoke.

Interestingly enough, it is assumed that Christian Science practitioners aren't really practicing medicine. They make no attempt at medical diagnosis, they prescribe no medication. They don't even touch their patients. They simply try to change their client's attitude toward disease by means of prayer. For the practitioner, diagnosis of the client's problem is really unimportant. The practitioner, you see, is trying to purge his client of a whole package of mortal error, sin and disease rather than a particular ailment "that by knowing the unreality of disease, sin, and death, you demonstrate the allness of God."[10]

The prayer of the Christian Scientist is not a prayer of petition. There is no appealing to God to heal a person. Instead, the practitioner makes an appeal to substitute the spiritual, the essence of good, which is the ultimate reality, for the "unreality" of disease. If this is successful, then healing occurs.

A Christian Science practitioner's entire training consists of two weeks of religious instruction. (Questionable qualifications, to put it mildly; remember Red Flag No. 9?) Yet the church doesn't limit the diseases its practitioners may treat. Nor does it require them to refer anyone for further treatment. They not only reject drugs, but they are also against pain-relieving measures such as hotpacks, enemas, and even back rubs. Still, spokesman Nathan Talbott contends that the testimonials published by the church, telling of people having been healed, is evidence enough of the practitioners' effectiveness.

A totally unbiased group, we're sure! (Another red flag.)

Most people would clearly put Christian Science into the category of alternative health care systems. Talbott disagrees. He says, "Christian Science is far from an alternative health care system. This evidence of healing and of the inner transformation that accompanies it has become as much a part of the daily experience of its adherents that they naturally turn to prayer in time of need."[11]

Is Christian Science really Christian? Absolutely not. Mary Baker Eddy claimed to speak in the name of Jesus, yet her teachings are in complete conflict with His. Is it really science? Not at all. Their methods belie any semblance to scientific methods.

Jesus warned us about people like Mary Baker Eddy. In Matthew 7:15–16 we read: "Beware of false prophets, who come to you in sheep's clothing, but inwardly they are ravenous wolves. You will know them by their fruits."

OTHER MIND-OVER-MATTER GROUPS

Other groups also exalt the mind in the healing process. The United Church of Religious Science (Science of Mind), founded by Ernest Holmes, teaches that "man controls the course of his life, his success or failure, his health or sickness, his happiness, boredom or misery, by mental processes which function according to a universal law.[12] Apply the principles of this law, and you can control it all. Of course, if you *fail* to apply the principles, you will lose all control. Science of Mind adherents believe the Bible to be just one of many sacred scriptures.

As for Jesus, this group claims that "any world teacher who helps mankind to be free from material, intellectual or emotional bondage is a spiritual savior." He's no more than a good example who allows us to affirm the divinity of us all. Sickness and health, they teach, is all a state of mind. So are heaven and hell. Like Christian Science, the group uses licensed practitioners, lay persons who have been trained to help people use the art and skill of "spiritual mind treatment" to solve problems and to cure illness.

The current public and private policies with regard to such groups should be a warning to those of us concerned about the inroads the alternative medicine movement is making in our society. Their practitioners are exempted from state licensing, although the Internal Revenue Service has been persuaded to allow sums paid to church practitioners to be deducted as medical expenses. The church has fought for and won exemptions from immunizations, prenatal blood testing, and metabolic testing of newborn babies. They have succeeded in having the Department of Health, Education, and Welfare place a religious immunity clause in the Code of Federal Regulations, effectively preventing in some cases prosecution of parents who withhold medical treatment from their children on the basis of religious beliefs.

With the precedent set, the way is paved for any New Age medical practice to have its particular health agenda recognized—depending, of course, on its lobbyists' success with their local legislatures or Congress.

Not all mind science health methods operate as overtly as these religions. Some call themselves science. Some insist they are nothing more than exercise, relaxation, or attempts to understand oneself. Let's look at some of these mind techniques and see what is behind each.

BIOFEEDBACK

Biofeedback is an American contribution to alternative health care. The holistic health movement loves to refer to biofeedback, because it seems to lend authenticity to their practices. Glance through almost any book on holistic medicine and you will find an inordinate number of references to biofeedback. Like hypnosis, biofeedback is frequently listed right alongside truly questionable practices.

Biofeedback consists of three basic operations. First, a particular physiologic response, such as heart rate, is detected and amplified, usually electronically. Second, this signal is converted into an easily understood form, such as a beeping electronic sound or a wavy line on a screen. And third, the transformed signal is immediately fed back to the patient—on a monitor, for instance.

To picture how this works, think of a patient lying in the intensive care unit, listening to his heart monitor beeping. As he concentrates on his heart rate, he becomes nervous. The beeping speeds up. The speeding up of his heart makes the patient more anxious than ever, and so the beeping gets still faster. Conversely, picture the same person practicing relaxation techniques. Through relaxation, he can actually learn to lower his heart rate.

At the center of biofeedback is the idea that people control their own physical responses. It is self therapy. This is what makes it so very attractive to those involved in alternative healing.

Many stories are told about the successes of biofeedback, and uncontrolled case studies are eagerly snatched up and used to substantiate particular health claims. Each is dramatic or sensational, sometimes both. Some reports are overtly biased. Some make patently wrong claims. Some are out and out fakes. Frequently a story will be told, then its successes generalized to make it seem to apply to other cases.

"It's proof!" proponents say. "This woman learned to control her migraine headaches. You can control your health problem, too, whatever it is."

It is a mistake to conclude that just because biofeedback worked for one person with one particular problem, biofeedback can work for almost any problem. It just doesn't happen that way.

Legitimate Uses of Biofeedback

Although biofeedback is far from the panacea for all ailments, it has proven its usefulness in a variety of disorders. As with other potentially helpful practices, to reject it out of hand because it is associated with the alternative health movement would rob patients of a potentially helpful treatment. This is as unfair and irrational as the claim that biofeedback is the answer for every problem. Biofeedback can stand up to scientific scrutiny and evaluation. Much in alternative medicine cannot.

Clinical feedback has been applied in only two basic types of practices: (1) Those where the physiological response the patient is trying to control is identified and directly related to the problem. An example of this is a patient with high blood pressure who is attempting to control a feedback signal, reflecting the level of his blood pressure. (2) Broader applications where the patient's complaint is caused by stress and she uses biofeedback for some physical response related to that stress. For example, a patient with high blood pressure works to decrease the muscle tension in her scalp muscles with biofeedback in order to reduce the stress, and thereby reduce her blood pressure.

The Alternative Approach

In alternative health, however, biofeedback is typically taught for general relaxation. As in other types of alternative health care, it often encourages the patient to achieve an altered state of consciousness. Nowhere in traditional biofeedback is there any such requirement.

Alternative health practitioners frequently quote three "basic principles" they claim underlie clinical biofeedback: (1) Any biological function can be monitored and amplified by electronic instruments. The information can be fed back to the person through any one of his five senses, and then can be regulated by that person. (2) Every change in the body is accompanied by an appropriate change in the mental or emotional state, either consciously or unconsciously. And every change in the mental or emotional state is accompanied by an appropriate change in the body. (3) Meditation and deep relaxation help to establish voluntary control by allowing the person to become aware of subliminal imagery, fantasies, and sensations.

Unscientific? Absolutely. But this doesn't deter alternative medicine advocates in the least.

DREAMWORK

Sigmund Freud called dreams "the royal road" to the unconscious. Carl Jung valued them as gateways to ever deeper levels of consciousness. That's why Jungian analysts spend so much time helping their patients interpret their dreams. Edgar Cayce, seer and prophet in the early 1900s, claimed to have done all his "work" while asleep. Dr. Bernie Siegel, whose work in alternative medicine we referred to earlier, says that the specific information and advice he gets out of dreams is incredible. He believes you can ask in a dream whether you should receive chemotherapy, and that you can dream the answer.

Could a dream really reveal the answer to such a vital question? Just what are the possibilities of our dream lives?

Bernie Siegel has been heavily influenced by Carl Jung, a foundation stone of the New Age. In both his books, Siegel quotes extensively from Jung and Jungian therapists. Dr. Siegel is so taken with dream therapy that he recommends keeping a dream diary where every night's dreams can be recorded. He calls this "an excellent way of getting back in touch with the unconscious."

Jonathan is a man who believes in getting in touch with his unconscious through his dream diary. "I didn't even realize I wasn't well," he says. "I found that out through my dreams." By interpreting his own dreams, Jonathan also discovered what he needed to do to improve his health (it all involved nutrition). He also found out when he was to marry and who was to be his wife.

"Dreams can't hurt," Siegel insists. They are "sent to help you." What he doesn't tell us is who sends them.

All of us dream. Scientists have done a great deal of research on dreams as a physical activity within the nervous system. Associated with rapid eye movement sleep (REM), dreams that most people recall occur about every three or four nights. Even animals are known to dream on a regular basis.

Some New Age healers suggest that the content of our dreams should influence our waking life. Taken too literally, this is a bit like living your life according to the fortune cookie you had for lunch. It's also a revival of pagan practices in ancient Greece, when priests and priestesses in over 600 temples of the Greek god of medicine advised about cures that dreams were said to hold.

Ancient Babylon and Egypt revered dreams as a window to the future and practiced dream divination. Dream books remain popular today as a means of guiding matters of health, work, and love. Modern day psychological theories of dreams as being the unfulfilled, repressed desires of the subconscious mind remain just that—theories. One would do well not to put too much stock in a particular dream, which is just as likely to be the result of poorly digested pepperoni pizza as to be some grand personal insight.

HYPNOSIS

"He called Barbara and me up on stage," Frank said of the nightclub entertainer who hypnotized him and his wife. "He put Barbara into a trance and took her back to when she was a little girl. She talked like a child, printed her name on the blackboard like a child, and cried when she was scolded. When it was my turn, Barbara told me later, I squawked and strutted around like a chicken. Everyone got a good laugh."

"I was hypnotized for the birth of each of my children," Janice said. "Each time it was a wonderful experience. I was awake and able to enjoy what was happening."

Hypnosis. No look at mind healing would be complete without discussing it.

The *Encyclopedia of Alternative Health Care* defines hypnosis as "the inducing of a trance-like state with heightened suggestibility or compliance." It isn't sleep, but it isn't quite an awake state either. Electroencephalograms of hypnotized persons show brain waves that are unlike both waking and sleeping brain waves.

Doctors and nurses in emergency rooms are well aware of the catatonic state in which people who have received an extreme shock can place themselves. This spontaneous, self-protective hypnotic state shields them from physical and emotional pain which would be overwhelming at the moment.

The biggest questions about hypnosis don't concern the procedure at all. Instead, our questions revolve around the state of heightened suggestibility. How will the unconscious mind perceive the suggestions given by the therapist? What will the reaction to these suggestions be?

Kathryn, a woman in her mid-thirties, was scheduled for a hysterectomy at the University of California Medical Center in Los Angeles. But she had a problem: She was extremely sensitive to anesthetics. The day before her surgery, she was approached by the chairman of the department of anesthesiology, who asked, "Would you consider being hypnotized for your surgery tomorrow?"

What a question! Kathryn thought. To her, hypnosis was more like witchcraft than modern medicine. The physician put Kathryn into a trance and demonstrated his technique. At his suggestion, the temperature of her left hand soared while her right hand turned blue with cold.

Realizing her options were few, Kathryn agreed to the hypnosis. No other anesthetic was given her. After the surgery, the physician gave her a post-hypnotic suggestion that kept her comfortable.

"It was a total success!" Kathryn told me. "I was awake during the surgery, and it didn't hurt at all. The doctor kept me informed on what was going on. When it was over, I felt fine."

Would she do it again?

"For me," she insists, "there *is* no other way."

It's Nothing New

Throughout history, hypnosis has reportedly been used for a variety of ailments, including dental extractions and anesthesia during childbirth. Today, one of the major problems with hypnosis is that it is practiced by so many people of varying abilities and purposes. Some, like the physician at UCLA, are trained medical personnel who use hypnosis for legitimate and beneficial purposes. Many others are therapists of questionable training who promise all kind of miracles. Then there are the stage artists who entertain by getting volunteers to bark like a dog or strut like a chicken.

Still, hypnosis is becoming more widely accepted as reports circulate of its effectiveness in dealing with such problems as obesity, tobacco addiction, and pain relief.

Dr. Eugene E. Levitt, secretary/treasurer of the American Board of Psychological Hypnosis and professor at the Indiana University School of Medicine, says, "Hypnosis is very, very good at pain control. That is one of its outstanding applied uses, particularly in pain due to clear-cut, bodily pathology (disease)."[13]

More and more medical uses for hypnosis are being discovered. In New Orleans, Dr. Dabney Ewin, a surgeon and psychiatrist who teaches hypnosis at Tulane University, uses it to treat widespread third degree burns. He believes this treatment can prevent inflammation, pain, and skin damage.[14]

Hypnosis is also increasingly becoming associated with

questionable practices, including past life regression therapy. Some promoters of hypnosis go so far as to suggest a person can increase her health, wealth, and wisdom in as little as one session with a hypnotherapist.

In 1958, the American Medical Association accepted hypnosis as a valid therapeutic technique. Since then, many psychiatrists, psychologists, doctors, lay counselors, and even ministers have added hypnosis to their repertoires of treatment methods for physical and emotional illness. Hypnosis, many claim, can help a therapist get at the root of a patient's problems more quickly than can traditional psychoanalysis.

Sounds good. The sooner the root cause is discovered, the sooner the patient can return to full health.

How Does It Work?

Some researchers believe that in some powerful way hypnosis distracts the subject from pain. Another theory is that during hypnosis the brain releases opiate-like pain killers called endorphins. Others believe it acts more through the emotions. But in fact, no one really knows for sure just how it works.

In hypnosis, the practitioner begins by putting his subject into a trance where she may experience various phenomena, such as "trance logic." In trance logic, she responds to specific suggestions. For instance, the hypnotist may give her a pencil and tell her it's a red-hot metal poker. Immediately she will react with pain and drop the pencil. Later the hypnotist will ask her, "Which did you see, a hot poker or a pencil?"

"A pencil," she answers. "But it felt red-hot. It burned my hand!"

Although not everyone is easy to hypnotize, anyone who is motivated and approached appropriately can learn to enter this trance state.

Sidney Petrie, in his book *What Modern Hypnotism Can do for You,* writes that hypnotism was practiced exclusively by witch doctors, Greek oracles, Persian Magi, and Hindu fakirs until as recently as two centuries ago. Interesting associations.

Before you decide to become involved with hypnosis, it is important to determine whether there is going to be any attempt to contact the unseen, non-material world. When hypnotism is combined with such things as Ouiji boards or automatic writing, it becomes a form of divination, something the Bible explicitly warns us to avoid (see Deut. 18:9–14).

Without a doubt, the company it keeps often calls hypnosis into question. A survey on the last page of a New Age magazine concerning New Age subjects listed hypnosis right alongside of astrology, crystal ball readings, witchcraft, tarot card readings, astro-projection, yoga, out-of-body experiences, and palm reading. The book *Witchcraft, Magic and Occultism,* by W. B. Crow, lists some of the occult sciences as witch doctors, druids and fairies, the black mass, the Kabalah, yoga, alchemy, and *hypnotism*. The book *Positive Living and Health,* by the editors of *Prevention* magazine, says in the opening sentence of a chapter on hypnotherapy: "Like alchemy and astrology, hypnosis once belonged to the world of the occult." They go on to add, "But, then, so did medicine." This is a clear, though unintentional, warning.

Who's in Control?

"I was afraid of hypnosis," Kathryn says, "because I was afraid I would be under someone else's control. Who knows what he would tell me to do?"

Physicians who work in the field of hypnotherapy agree with Dr. Jeanine LaBaw's answer to this concern. A Denver physician who works with hypnosis and pain, Dr. LaBaw says, "You totally maintain your own control. You won't do anything immoral. You won't take your clothes off and cluck like a chicken unless you happen to like being the life of the party." She goes on to say that although many people think that in a trance a person will do anything that the hypnotist wants them to do, such isn't true of real hypnosis.[15]

Surprisingly, we think that one of the best warning statements about hypnosis comes from Kristin Olsen, author of the

---

Encyclopedia of Alternative Health Care: "Hypnosis is like a gun. It's not the tool itself, but the operator who makes it dangerous. It is the state of altered consciousness which makes an individual vulnerable to suggestion from a hypnotist."

Although hypnosis puts a patient in a vulnerable position, and although it can possibly lead to a feeling of dependency on the therapist, no training or credentials are generally required for those who would act as hypnotherapists. So, in the end, discernment is our own responsibility. If the purpose is a legitimate medical one, then hypnosis may indeed be called for. But if the purpose is to enter an altered state of consciousness in order to practice a form of the occult, we should steer clear of it.

We also need to ask a few questions. Is the practitioner a licensed physician or certified by some professional group? Is he or she associated with a medical school? A wise person should certainly check the credentials, background, and the general philosophy of any person he would allow to take control of his unconscious mind.

Yet even in a proper setting, hypnosis can be misused. It is not an innocuous plaything to be taken lightly.

Without a doubt, many aspects of hypnosis can be beneficial to a patient. It makes no sense to forbid its use entirely just because it can be invoked to enter an altered state of consciousness. It's not the altered state of consciousness the Bible speaks against. It's the practices that can take place in that state.

TRANSCENDENTAL MEDITATION

A long-haired, white-bearded man sits gazing serenely straight ahead. He is Maharishi Mahesh Yogi. You can see his picture in almost any newspaper, on flyers pasted on bulletin boards of college campuses, in tabloids, and in magazines. He offers free introductory lectures on Transcendental Meditation (TM), which he founded. The flyers assure us this is "not a religion, philosophy or life-style."

Sounds pretty good. But let's take a closer look.

Austin, Texas, is a pretty important place to the Maharishi. The town where we live is being billed by his group as a Nirvana for the '90s. A newspaper article reported:

> Following a master plan touted by the Maharishi Mahesh Yogi (his followers) set their sights on creating "a New Age style community southwest of Austin that will be known as the City of Immortals." These visionaries have conceived of a world wide movement fashioned of "harmonious, largely self-contained residential areas that are free of pollution, crime and anxiety." Developers state they intend to establish a community health facility designed to "balance the whole person—mind, body, behavior and environment. The goal is to prevent disease and promote perfect health and longevity creating a disease-free individual and disease-free society.[16]

But apparently not even the Maharishi is immune from financial pressure, since a more recent newspaper report says the "City of Immortals" will have to wait until the Texas economy improves a bit.

Even medical literature is now starting to refer to meditation. An article in *The Family Practice News,* July 15, 1989, tells of a family practice resident who contracted cancer. In an editorial the physician states that after her diagnosis and initial treatment she did an elective on healing. It was "good because it gave me a framework to do all the work I had to do. I started doing yoga three times a week and meditation just to get grounded again."

Her perspective had changed, the physician insisted. "We should not be trying to cure the patient," she said, "but to empower the patient to enable him to cure himself." As a result of her experiences with alternative healing, she wrote: "Now I realize there is a whole other side of healing—an exciting spiritual side."

Spiritual side? But the Maharishi's poster said this was definitely not religious. And who is this Maharishi anyway?

Maharishi Mahesh Yogi was a Hindu monk who brought TM

to the United States in 1959. He is known not by his name, but by the title he assumed for himself. Maharishi means "great seer" or "great sage." Mahesh is a family name, and Yogi means "Master of Yoga." The so-called Maharishi follows his own guru—Guru Dev, a "divine teacher." It was from him that the Maharishi developed his teaching that later became TM.

Where It All Started

The Maharishi claims that TM's roots go back thousands of years to Krishna, then to Buddha—though the Maharishi claims the Buddhists have distorted the teaching. The teaching was restored by a Hindu teacher in A.D. 800, although it was confined primarily to a few Hindus and Yogis living in Himalayan caves. This changed when Guru Dev came into the full knowledge of the teaching and passed it on to Maharishi Mahesh Yogi.

The Maharishi began to hold introductory lectures on college campuses in the United States, and he founded a student organization he called the Students' International Meditation Society. Within six years of its formation, SIMS claimed to have more than 10,000 members in the United States.

Maharishi Yogi really hit the big time when he was introduced to the Beatles. Photos of them with him generated an enormous interest. It was in Madison Square Garden that the Maharishi revealed his plan for permanent world peace. What the world really needed, he said, was one meditation center staffed by one teacher for every 100,000 people. But as the show biz and musical stars turned their attention away from Maharishi Yogi, the initial enthusiasm for TM began to subside.

In the 1960s the Maharishi was open about TM's religious heritage. A true visionary, he advised in his book *Transcendental Meditation,* that "It seems for the present that this transcendent, deep meditation should be made available to the peoples through the agencies of government . . . health, education, social welfare and justice."[17]

Now, this posed a very real problem here in the United States. We have a constitutional prohibition against government being involved in religion.

Never one to be deterred, the Maharishi reoriented his movement. He explained that what happened during the practice of meditation was actually a physiologic event which he called "the science of creative intelligence."

In 1970, Maharishi Yogi's devoted follower, Jerry Jarvis, got Science of Intelligence scheduled as a credit course at Stanford University. Now the Maharishi really had something. Suddenly TM was just another self-help technique for dealing with the stresses of modern life.

In 1972, an article written by Dr. Robert Wallace and Dr. Herbert Benson appeared in *The Scientific American*. The doctors described the physiological effects they observed from the practice of TM: a state of rest marked by physiological changes such as decreased oxygen consumption, lowered heart rate, increased skin resistance, and the identification of the brain's alpha waves. This was to become a major force in establishing the credibility of TM's new image as a non-religious, scientific approach to the problems of today.

The Master Plan

It was the Maharishi's plan to teach TM to the entire world. The group incorporated as an educational organization, and the Maharishi Yogi outlined for the world seven goals he claimed could be reached by practicing TM: (1) Develop the full potential of the individual. (2) Improve governmental achievement. (3) Realize the highest ideal of education. (4) Solve the problems of crime and all behavior that brings unhappiness to the family of man. (5) Maximize the intelligent use of the environment. (6) Bring fulfillment to the economic aspirations of the individual. (7) Achieve the spiritual goals of mankind during this generation.

By 1975, the United States government had funded seventeen research grants for TM projects. People were joining the movement at the rate of 30,000 a month. Two books on TM had made the best seller list.

The introductory lectures claimed that TM was simply a scientific technique that anybody could learn. The practice could relieve stress and lower blood pressure. In fact, it would provide a variety of other benefits as well, including increased sexual performance and enjoyment. However, they reiterated, TM was *not* a religion, nor was it a religious practice.

Yet a prospective meditator had to undergo an initiation ceremony for which he must remove his shoes before entering a candlelighted, incense-filled room. There he had to place a flower offering on a new, clean, white handkerchief in front of a picture of Guru Dev. All the while an initiator would sing a "puja" hymn and bow and kneel before the picture of Dev, instructing the initiate to do the same. The purpose of this initiation was to give the new meditator his mantra, a secret word essential for the practice of TM.

Not religious? The entire practice of TM revolves around letting the mantra "dwell" in one's consciousness. TM instructors claim that the mantras are meaningless sounds with nothing but vibrational qualities beneficial to the nervous system. Other TMers disagree. They insist that a mantra is a sacred text, that the words are holy and indestructible, and that when properly repeated, a mantra could—according to Hindu beliefs—produce miracles. Although the Maharishi said the mantras were assigned according to unique, personal characteristics, ex-TM teachers report they were given a short list of mantras and instructed to dispense them to the initiates by categories of age and sex.

Even the secular news media recognized TM for what it was—a religious practice. *Psychology Today* called it "Clearly a revival of ancient Indian Brahmanism and Hinduism whose origins lie in the ancient texts—Vedas, Upanishads and Bhagavad-Gita; the teachings of the Buddha."[18]

Eventually, public and private high schools with adult education programs began to offer courses in TM. Public high schools in New Jersey obtained a $40,000 grant from the department of Health, Education, and Welfare for experimental TM classes in the 1975-76 school year. This prompted a legal challenge of TM's "non-religious" claim, and the organization was sued by three non-profit organizations and several New Jersey taxpayers to prevent the courses from being taught. It violated the constitutional requirement of separation of church and state, they insisted. The court agreed. The judge remarked, "Despite TM's objections, religious concepts did not become less religious just because they are taught as philosophy of science." TM was barred from public schools.

The issue is really one of informed choice. If, after careful consideration you decide that you should become a Hindu or follow the teachings of Buddha, that is certainly your choice. But don't allow yourself to be tricked into becoming involved in TM so you can lower your blood pressure. A good diet and a nap will do the same for you, without risking the loss of your immortal soul.

Hindus have no difficulty absorbing other religious teachings. They believe every man is free to worship God in his own way, that in the end all roads lead to the same One God. Jesus disagreed. In John 14:6 He said, "I am the way, the truth, and the life. No one comes to the Father except through Me." In Matthew 7:13–14 He said, "Enter by the narrow gate; for wide is the gate and broad is the way that leads to destruction, and there are many who go in by it. Because narrow is the gate and difficult is the way which leads to life, and there are few who find it."

YOGA

Everyone has heard of yoga. It conjures up visions of extremely flexible men and women sitting in unusual poses, doing seemingly impossible stretching exercises for the sake of their health. Generally we think of it as a form of exercise. The synopsis for the Hatha Yoga class at the University of Texas at Austin states that yoga was developed as a science with specific methods for bettering the total well-being of an individual. Hatha Yoga, it says, consists of "postures" that work on the major physiological systems.

Some people insist that yoga has actually healed them of serious illness, and they are quick to tell their stories to back up their claims. An article in the November/December 1989 issue of *Yoga Journal* tells about a fellow by the name of Eric Small, who claims he had multiple sclerosis (MS), a degenerative nerve disease for which there is no known cure. For the past seven years he says he has kept the disease in remission through yoga. Says Mr. Small, "Hatha Yoga is effective where physical therapy isn't in that you become your own teacher."

That sounds pretty good. But the fact is that only a small number of MS cases actually progress to complete disability. By nature, the disease is characterized by remissions and recurrences. Mr. Small's insistence that his remission is due to yoga sounds like wishful thinking.

A Philosophy Without Sin

Yoga is based on a Hindu philosophy, which denies the reality of sin: "It is a sin to call anyone a sinner. It is a standing libel on human nature. Vedanta does not believe in sin, only error, and the greatest error is to think you are weak."[19]

We see quite a different philosophy laid out in the Bible. In order to stamp out the concept of sin there, you'd have to delete large portions of the Holy Scriptures. One of the first sections to go would be Paul's writings in Romans where he says in 6:23, "For the wages of sin is death, but the gift of God is eternal life in Christ Jesus our Lord." You would also have to erase the person of Jesus Christ, since He came to earth to save us from our sins. In 1 Timothy 1:15 Paul writes that "Christ Jesus came into the world to save sinners."

The goal of advanced yoga students is to attain their highest possible degree of physical, mental, and spiritual integration, and ultimately to reach union with Brahma, the Hindu concept of the cosmic God. Although many in our country engage in yoga classes simply for exercise, it is a fact that yoga migrated to the west as a spiritual discipline. Vegetarianism and nonviolence are two additional key elements of yoga philosophy.

Even though the practice of yoga focuses on a series of stretching exercises, breathing practices, and meditation to reach a state of peace and harmony, this physical discipline is merely a means to an end. The goal is to reach the state of Samadhi, or a state of union with God.

Is It Scientific?

Does yoga have scientific validity? Some claim it can unclog arteries and control high blood pressure. Well, there are many ways to control high blood pressure. Merely losing as little as ten pounds is reported to lower the diastolic pressure in an average person by ten millimeters of mercury. Add to that a regular aerobic exercise program, and blood pressure certainly can be reduced. Or a person can cut down on the salt or fat in his diet.

We do have a report in a reputable medical journal sponsored by the Aerospace Medical Association of one aviator who, through the use of relaxation techniques, was able to control his high blood pressure. Other studies from medical colleges in India claim yoga helped in such cases as asthma and blood coagulation.

Should the fact that yoga apparently produces isolated physiologic effects suggested that it should be widely accepted? We have to question this. Anyone—especially any Christian—entering into the practice of yoga should do so with his eyes wide open to the Hindu philosophy underlying the practice.

The Himalayan International Institute of Yoga Science and Philosophy in Honesdale, Pennsylvania, is a retreat for yoga studies. They describe themselves as "a non-profit organization devoted to teaching holistic health, yoga and meditation as means to foster the personal growth of the individual and the betterment of society." They view the institute as "building a bridge between the perennial truths of the East and the modern discoveries of the West." There are training programs for counselors and therapists, nurses, and dietitians, and a seminar for physicians.

The back page of the Himalayan Institute quarterly consists of an advertisement for special courses held at the Institute specifically for health care professionals. These include "New Perspectives on Health" aimed at nurses, and "The Principle and Practice of Holistic Medicine," a seminar for physicians. Clearly it is the intention of the Institute to recruit nurses and doctors into the ranks of yoga practitioners.

More and more, their effort is successful.

Positive thinking is potent medicine. Faith, too, is exceedingly powerful. Most of us will readily agree that there is a difference between scientific fact and out-and-out mumbo-jumbo. The question is, Where is the dividing line? The answer depends on who you ask.

You might start by asking Matthew Swan's parents.

Chapter Seven

MAY THE FORCE BE WITH YOU

Energy Manipulating Therapies

"**S**tar Wars was the best movie to come along in years," the principal told a large group of parents assembled in the auditorium of a Christian school in Southern California. "The Force, you see, is God."

Is it? Not likely. According to the movie's New Age makers, the Force is "universal energy."

Universal energy? you may ask. What's that? Good question.

IS UNIVERSAL ENERGY RELIGIOUS?

Paul Reisser, M.D., author of *New Age Medicine,* identifies certain characteristics of universal energy as defined by practitioners of holistic medicine. (1) Universal energy is the basic fabric of everything in the universe. (2) Disease results from a blockage or imbalance in the flow of energy in the body. (3) Universal energy can be activated or channeled by a healer, and may be used either constructively or destructively. (4) Alterations in universal energy are the basis for all events that have previously been called supernatural or miraculous. (5) Universal energy is what religions have called God.

143

Like the California principal, some Christians view this "energy" to be either God or a creation of God. But is it actually from God at all? Does it even exist, or might it have other deceptive purposes?

W. Brugh Joy, M.D., is a Fellow of the American College of Physicians and a Phi Beta Kappa graduate from the University of Southern California and USC School of Medicine. In *Joy's Way: A Map for the Transformation Journey,* Dr. Joy wrote an introduction to the potentials for healing with body energies. What he prescribes is a visualization technique he calls "command therapy" to achieve healing. This is preliminary to the introduction of his readers to body energy fields called chakras.

The term *chakras* refers to the seven centers of psychic spiritual energy from the yoga teachings of Hinduism. Supposedly located like little spiritual batteries along a person's spine, various alternative healing techniques are said to manipulate the energy in these chakras for healing purposes. The claim that these New Age healing methods have no spiritual effect on the person is about as likely as someone eating a hot dog at a rock concert without realizing the music is playing.

Claiming that disturbances in chakras lead to ill health, Joy believes that mental imagery can realign these energy disturbances. Again and again we will see that alternative approaches overlap. Much like Christian Science, Unity, and Science of Mind religions, which all practice the power of mind over matter, Dr. Joy said of his healing energies, "Mental imagery is the basis of mental healing."

With patients in an altered state of consciousness (once again, Red Flag No. 11!), Joy claims the healer may practice healing techniques in a transfer of energy from healer to subject. That such practices are occultic in nature and lead to interaction with an unseen world of supernatural forces is clear when Dr. Joy describes fields of energy that can appear to take on the form of a human, an animal, an angelic being, a demon or even an Inner Teacher. Recognizing the apprehension his followers must feel when this happens in some altered state of consciousness, he attempts to ease those fears by explaining that these entities are only projections of people's minds. If a thought form materializes as a demon, a person need only dissolve the thought form and the demon would disappear.

Interesting concept. But if demons are simply imaginary ghosts conjured up by our own thoughts, why, after Jesus cast a demon out of a man, would Luke write, "For with authority and power He [Jesus] commands the unclean spirits, and they come out" (Luke 4:36).

Universal energy is said to be activated and channeled by a healer. Acupuncture needles or some other form of stimulation at specific acupuncture points are supposed to cause energy to flow more evenly, or to adjust the flow of energy, or to relieve blockages in energy flow. Alterations in universal energy, proponents insist, are the basis for all events which have been called supernatural or miraculous. Based on this, an invisible and undetectable energy source provides alternative health groups with a ready explanation for their supposedly miraculous powers of clairvoyance, psychokinesis, and medical miracles.

Universal Energy goes by different names in different cultures. In China it's Chi, while in Japan it is Kai. In India it is known as prana. D. D. Palmer, founder of Chiropractic, and a great believer in universal energy, called it "the Innate." Dr. Bernie Siegel, in *Love, Medicine & Miracles,* says this energy is God. But let me assure you that David, the ancient king of Israel, was not crying out to some energy force when he wrote in Psalm 69:1, "Save me, O God!"

By their very definition, therapies based on the theory of energy manipulation should cause Red Flag No. 2 (our warning against claims to use psychic power, chapter 4), to fly high. Let's look at some of the names under which we will find energy manipulation.

ACUPUNCTURE

One of the most popular forms of energy manipulation is acupuncture, a well-known practice in Chinese medicine. Its proponents use it to stimulate points on the body's surface to affect physiologic changes, either in the whole body or in specific areas. Stimulation is achieved by inserting extremely fine needles into specific points on the skin.

Sometimes practitioners also apply heat. This process, called moxabustion, involves a small moistened cone of dried plants and herbs which is placed on the acupuncture point, burned directly on the skin, then crushed to form a blisterlike cover. Heat generated from an electric light or a laser probe is sometimes used to stimulate the points. There may also be an application of pressure in the form of massage or acupressure.

Taoist Roots

Today acupuncturists are in nearly every major city in the United States. Many patients who accept the treatments have no idea that the philosophies behind acupuncture are firmly rooted in the religious tenents of Taoism, a difficult to understand ancient Oriental philosophy with religious implications. In his book *The Tao of Leadership,* John Heider says: "Tao is the single unifying principle underlying all creation." Others have described Tao as the "invisible, inaudible, unnameable, undiscussable, inexpressible."[1] The principles of acupuncture are based upon such a foundation of intellectual quicksand.

One of the recognized textbooks from which Chinese medicine is supposedly descended is the *Yellow Emperors Classic of Internal Medicine,* a volume said to have been written in 762 A.D. In the introduction to this book it is noted: "This combination is in matter of fact the only way in which early Chinese medical thinking could be expressed, for medicine was but a part of philosophy and religion, both of which propounded oneness with nature." Chinese medicine is based on Taoism.

Although the Taoists see this universal energy flow as uniting all of nature, they are also interested in the concept of polarity, the yin and yang. Yang is supposedly positive, expansive, masculine, light, big, having the nature of heaven, of day, of the left side as opposed to the right, of the surfaces of an object, of wood, and of fire. Yin, on the other hand, is negative, contractive, feminine, dark, small, having the nature of earth, of night, of the right side, and the interior of an object. Taoists believe all substances are a mixture of these qualities, and that when they are balanced properly the body will be healthy. In fact, Chinese medical doctors classify the organs of the body as yin and yang, hollow ones being yang and solid ones being yin.

A classic element of Chinese medicine is pulse diagnosis. Chinese doctors believe energy imbalances are reflected in changes of superficial pulses. As a physician, when I feel the pulse in my patients' wrists, I get clues. I'm primarily interested in the rate and the rhythm of the heartbeat: Is it fast or slow, regular or irregular? Chinese doctors, on the other hand, believe that through pulse diagnosis—which they say requires years of practice—they can get detailed information regarding the functioning of various organs and just where energy deficiencies lie. They record twelve different pulses, six on each wrist, each of which correlates to the bodily function of a specific organ system. Never mind that there is not a bit of scientific basis for this.

Traditional Chinese therapists follow many other rules. For instance, they will not perform acupuncture if the outside temperature exceeds the body temperature. (This would be difficult in the southwest. I wonder if acupuncturists here in Texas close down their offices during the summer months.) Traditional therapists cannot perform acupuncture during the full moon or during lightning storms. (What happens if a person gets sick during such times? Too bad.)

Chinese medicine has grown into a fad since a *New York Times* reporter underwent an emergency appendectomy during an official visit by Americans to China, shortly after the communist revolution. His story of how acupuncture relieved his postoperative pain created a great deal of interest and a demand for acupuncture in the United States.

Scientific Problems

One problem arises from the number of acupoints on the human body. A traditional number is 365, based astrologically on the number of days in the year, and spread along fourteen meridians or energy channels. Each point corresponds to a specific area of the body and is related to a particular internal organ. By stimulating these points, the balance of the flow of energy circulating through these meridians is supposedly manipulated, adjusted, and freed from blockage.

Skeptics have a question: How can two separate and opposite problems be treated by the same acupuncture point, such as the zusanli point, which is the treatment spot for both diarrhea and constipation? Good question. We've heard no plausible answer.

Many within scientific medicine strongly disagree with the claims of acupuncture. Dr. Charles A. Fager, chairman emeritus of the Department of Neurosurgery of the Lahey Clinic in Burlington, Massachusetts, says:

> There is not the slightest shred of evidence to show that acupuncture produces any real physiological changes. . . . There is no physiologic reason why if you stick a needle in somebody's ear, a pain in the small of the back will go away. The anesthesia is simply hypnosis. Acupuncture is basically a form of deception and fraud and should be against the law.[2]

According to acupuncture theory, insufficiency in one organ would also lead to a similar insufficiency of energy in another organ. For example, an excess of energy in the liver would lead to an excess of energy in the heart. Certainly there is no scientific basis for these relationships. (Red Flag No. 8, "Explanations that don't make sense," springs up.)

Traditionally, the primary role of acupuncture has been the prevention of disease by maintaining a person's good health. The Chinese believed the manipulation of the energy flow kept them healthy. Only as a secondary resort would they use acupuncture to actually cure physical problems. In this country, however, treatment has become the primary role of acupuncture.

It is difficult to assess present western practices of acupuncture, for seldom is the Chinese technique of diagnosis used to determine what acupuncture treatment is really needed. Most scientific evaluations of the technique now use a formula treatment—that is, when anyone has a certain problem, the same specific acupuncture points are stimulated. Treatment is not at all personalized.

The fact that it isn't possible to perform accurate studies makes it even more difficult to assess how well acupuncture works. It could be argued that while a skilled acupuncturist always knows which points are being treated, an unskilled therapist—one who is simply told to insert needles in specific sites—can't be counted upon to accurately locate the points.

Studies that have been done have yielded confusing results. In one experiment, bronchial patients who were treated at the acupuncture points appropriate for migraine headaches did better than those treated at the points appropriate for bronchial asthma. No one was able to explain why this happened.

Although anesthesia by acupuncture has been discussed a great deal, its use is subject to question. Most evaluations for acupuncture anesthesia have either been published in China or in acupuncture journals such as *The American Journal of Chinese Medicine*. Still, a large number of surgeries have been performed in which acupuncture was purportedly the only anesthesia. These range from tooth extractions to appendectomies to Cesarean sections to surgeries for breast cancer to gastrectomies (removal of the stomach).

How Does It Work?

Some American researchers feel that acupuncture works by releasing endorphins—natural painkillers produced by the body. Others believe it is simply a placebo effect; the power of belief is often very strong in acupuncture subjects. Some believe it is the power of suggestion, or hypnosis, which causes the physiologic changes. Others are more in agreement with the universal energy theory, although some prefer to call it "body electricity." Some have referred to the gate theory, which proposes that there are neuropathway gates along the spinal cord en route to the brain, and that through acupuncture the gates may be closed, thus blocking the pain message.

While no one seems to know for sure just how acupuncture does work, there is no denying it is effective in some patients. Of course, so are placebos. To further complicate matters, acupuncture is frequently both unpredictable and unreliable.

Today in our country, acupuncturists are attempting to cure various problems such as obesity and smoking. An article was published in *The American Journal of Medicine* which reported that acupuncture needle holes placed in the ear were effective against smoking addiction. Unfortunately, the study was uncontrolled. Also, in addition to the acupuncture the patients were given anti-smoking indoctrination. So, how could you possibly tell which therapy helped?

According to the authors, the "anti-smoking" ear point was discovered by chance when two overweight nurses were treated for obesity by a needle in the ear and both suddenly stopped smoking. If this was the case, then the anti-obesity point is identical to the anti-smoking point. One would expect that overweight smokers so treated could then always lose weight. Yet this doesn't happen.

An Even Better Question

Our usual question revolves around whether or not acupuncture really works and how we can use it. But we may be neglecting an even more important question: Given its heavy emphasis on Taoism, what effect might acupuncture-type treatments have on patients' belief system? What effect might it have on therapists?

It is also important to recognize that *treating* a disorder is not the same as *curing* it. Acupuncturists may indeed treat, but there is no evidence they can cure. It alarms me that many claim they can "treat" unidentified growths and masses. What if that growth turned out to be cancer? Being treated with acupuncture before a proper and correct diagnosis has been made could be a deadly mistake.

According to the New England School of Acupuncture (NESA), social, political, religious, and spiritual forces worked together to evolve into what we know today as acupuncture. Religion is a heavy element. There is no way a student can attend NESA in Watertown, Massachusetts, without being heavily influenced by the Taoist aspects of yin and yang and the balancing of vital energy force. In their classes the major philosophies of Confucianism, Taoism, Monism, Legalism, and Yin/Yang theory are all examined.

In most states, acupuncturists don't need a license to practice. Unlicensed, they are beyond the reach of any regulatory agency. That's not a reassuring thought when someone is poking you full of needles in this age of AIDS. With no license to lose, they needn't worry about not being able to practice, so the public remains unprotected.

Acupuncture? It has not been shown to be universally effective, and it may be damaging. Let the patient beware!

APPLIED KINESIOLOGY

If nurses have embraced therapeutic touch, chiropractors have done the same with a technique known as applied kinesiology. Kinesiology itself is the legitimate study and science of muscular motion. But what we are talking about here is definitely not a legitimate science.

Applied kinesiology was originated in the 1960s by a chiropractor named George Goodheart. By combining the concept of "innate intelligence" with the Eastern religious concept of energy, Goodheart came up with the idea that weak muscles would reflect back the condition of all the various organs of the body via the "Chi meridians." To him, muscle spasm was not so much a problem as was muscle weakness.

Goodheart took standard muscle testing techniques from physical therapy texts and combined them with Chinese concepts of energy flow. From this he produced a work entitled *Applied Kinesiology Research Manuals*. In it, the innate intelligence he affirmed was described as a spiritual intelligence that runs through the body and is connected to the universal intelligence through the nervous system. Does this sound familiar?

How Is It Supposed To Work?

John Thie, a chiropractor in Pasadena, California, wrote *Touch For Health,* a book that has become one of the most popular manuals of applied kinesiology. Thie's book consists primarily of diagrams of muscle tests and treatments. Its theoretical groundwork is stated in its opening pages: "The innate intelligence that runs the body is connected to universal intelligence that runs the world, so each person is plugged into the universal intelligence through the system." Thie relates this to classical chiropractic, which is said to clear the communication system between the nerves and the body.

With the claims of manipulated universal intelligence, we begin to detect an overlap into the religious aspects of Eastern mysticism.

Thie's book claims that certain muscles have special relationships with various internal organs. Never mind that these relationships have no basis in traditional anatomy; this is "chiropractic acupuncture."

Practitioners of applied kinesiology require no real training. All they need is their handy-dandy diagram of deficiency points, a trusting patient, and a picture of a man standing, with multiple points indicated on him—a point on the cheek for potassium, another on the center of the chest for iodine, and so on.

Two different points around the figure's belly button have the same elements—magnesium and manganese. How, you might ask, can the body tell the difference between these two elements? Good question. The best answer the practitioner has to offer is that she says out loud what it is she is testing for. If she says, "Now I'm testing for magnesium" as she touches the point on the belly button and does the muscle testing, then, we are told, her "brain will know the difference."

Ludicrous, you say? Totally unscientific? Makes absolutely no sense? (Red Flag No. 8.)

The most popular muscles tested in applied kinesiology are the deltoids (on the outside of the shoulders) and the finger muscles.

"He had me lie down and hold my arm straight out," Kate told me in describing the chiropractor who tested her. "He told me not to let him push it down. Then he put one bottle of pills after another on my chest and pushed on my arm. If I could resist him, he said I didn't need that supplement. If he could push my arm down, he said my body needed the pills."

Sometimes, a person doesn't even need to be there for the practitioner to test and prescribe. A full-time Christian worker told me he was encouraged by a woman in his church, an herbalist, to come to her shop. "I can help you with your health problems," she told him.

When he went to see her, he was amazed to find that she wanted to prescribe the herbs through muscle testing. Now, my friend is a large man and the woman is quite small. Physically, they couldn't manage this testing procedure. "No problem," she said, and proceeded to call in a proxy. She placed the proxy's hands on my friend's outstretched arms, then read the muscle weakness through the proxy.

My friend was skeptical, to say the least.

"It's just proving that the universal energy is flowing from you to the proxy and on to me," the herbalist told him. Somehow this makes perfect sense to someone who subscribes to the concept of universal energy.

One with the Universe

To really understand these "energies of the universe" which "take form in the individual," Thie said, "we must remember that we are all one with the universe, with the Universal Energy. When this energy is highly concentrated, we call it matter. Our bodies are that matter. Therefore, our bodies are literally this Universal Energy in some of its various forms."[3] What a clear example of New Age philosophy in the form of alternative health care! The universe is all energy, you're energy, we are all one. This energy is the essence of God. Therefore, we are God.

You are God. But there is a major problem with this reasoning. Whether it is New Age or Old Testament in the Garden of Eden, only Satan teaches that we are God's equal and worthy of the same praise we give Him.

The nature of the patient/doctor relationship implicitly involves a kind of trust. Along with this goes a willingness to submit to the healer's suggestions. Yet it is dangerous for any of us to passively accept this "submissive patient" stance. It can easily result in being duped medically and led astray spiritually.

Manipulation of universal energy is nothing but esoteric occultism, no matter how nice, or professional, or "Christian" the practitioner may be.

CRYSTALS

A young woman with long, flowing hair, a brightly colored shirt, faded jeans, and two crystal pendants around her neck walked into a health food store. She had a little boy of no more than a year and a half balanced on her hip. With her husband beside her, she hurried over to where a whole array of crystals were displayed on the counter. There were crystal pendants, crystal dust, crystal chips, large sparkling crystals on stands, crystals of every shape, size, and hue.

The young mother carefully rummaged through the display as the boy on her hip coughed and sniffled and rubbed his runny nose.

"This one?" her husband asked as he handed her a pendant.

"Too big," she replied. "It's almost the size of yours." She pointed to the large crystal he wore around his neck.

The young woman picked up a smaller one and held it up to the child. "It doesn't feel right," she said as she put it back.

The clerk came over and asked if she could be of help.

"I think my baby has a cold," the young woman explained. "He's having trouble breathing. I want to buy a crystal to get him well."

Crystals are everywhere. They are worn as jewelry and displayed as decorative prisms. They are displayed on desks and hung from car mirrors. A five-year-old patient of mine told me about her crystal and its power to heal. I had an AIDS patient who kept a large crystal quartz beside his bed. There are reports of nurses hanging crystals on I-V poles above their patients' beds in the intensive care unit.

Don't think this is just a practice of kooks. Crystals are fast becoming an accepted part of our mainstream society. Little old ladies are using them. Kids are using them. Church people are using them. Everyone seems to be doing it. And this tends to lend still more credibility to crystal power. Under the influence of New Agers, "pet rocks" have given way to "prayer rocks."

What's the Purpose?

A recent article on crystals in *Omni* magazine tells how various people use them. A marketing consultant in Philadelphia uses them to get rid of headaches, to help her house plants grow, and to increase the efficiency of her refrigerator. A Texas rancher uses them to keep flies away from his cattle. An optician in Pittsburgh, who practices metaphysical counseling and healing, regularly uses crystals and other stones. In the center of his office, suspended from the ceiling, is a large quartz crystal which he claims filters out all the bad vibrations left in the room by the aliens. It routes this negative energy to a crystal-tipped grounding rod in the basement.

At a New Age fair billed as a "cosmic rodeo" here in Austin, a variety of crystal vendors displayed an assortment of rocks that would impress any rock hound. "Touch them," the vendors urged. "Pick them up. Feel the vibrations. Find the one that works for you." Some suggested I try drinking juice mixed with ground up crystal powder. "Put this in your refrigerator," one told me. "It will accelerate the cooling and reduce your electric bill." Suggested another, "Attach this one to the carburetor in your car. It'll save you gas."

A young woman with an earnestness in her eyes and a large

crystal pendant around her neck told me, "It protects me. When I wear it, I have a circle of power around me. It keeps me safe."

The crystal therapy fad may well come and go, just as other fads do, but according to Russell Chandler, author of *Understanding the New Age:*

> The fallout of New Age thinking and its impact is going to be around for a long time. Many of its subtleties have penetrated the entire culture. It's very attractive and seductive, promising quick spirituality. Its eclectic appeal resonates with a lot of people in our pluralistic society.[4]

According to the New Age concept, the way crystals work is that a minute energy field pervades the entire known universe, including every piece of earth, and especially crystals.

Religious Aspects

When Christians hear people who are involved in such things as crystals using words like Christianity and Christ, and hear them making references to love and goodness and God, they begin to think it's all okay. It isn't.

Crystal therapy has a close relationship with the occult. If you doubt it, consider the words of Gary Fleck, one of the country's leading crystal suppliers. A miner by trade, Fleck was drawn into the New Age movement through his love of crystals, an affection he developed as a child growing up in Arizona. Fleck says that one day he led an expedition of crystal lovers into a mine in Arizona so everyone could offer special prayers with their crystals. Upon arriving in the cavern, each pilgrim lit a candle. Suddenly, an "angel" appeared to him.

Almost everyone in the group saw the angel, Fleck insists. She identified herself as Sabatina, a spirit of the inner earth. Then she put her hands on Fleck's head and began to pronounce the role of crystals in human destiny. Fleck tells us he felt as if he were a conduit for a being. He translated the angel's words to an awestruck prayer circle.

What Sabatina supposedly had to say was that crystals and gems "are here to teach and heal. If you want to learn what they can teach and how they can heal, then ask the crystals themselves. They are alive. They should be treated as friends." She went on to say that crystals were only one path to a higher consciousness. "When you go fishing, you use a shiny lure. Crystals are shiny lures as well, and they can serve to hook people on the idea of reaching for a higher consciousness."[5]

That's exactly what a physical therapist working at a local health spa told me when I asked her about the crystal obelisk around her neck. "I like the way it looks," she replied.

Why does my AIDS patient have his crystal? Because his friends brought it over and he likes "the way crystals look."

The lure is there. The involvement with the occult is right around the corner. It's all straight from the words of Sabatina, Fleck's spirit of the inner earth.

Spiritual Seduction

There is another side to crystal healing. *Inside The New Age Nightmare,* by Randall N. Baer, tells the story of a professional New Age teacher, holistic health practitioner, and holistic activist who became renowned both in "crystal power" and in New Age philosophy.

Baer was brought up in a middle class home, his father a medical doctor and his mother a nurse. As a teenager he was entranced with the Eastern mystical concepts depicted on the television show "Kung Fu," and he read many books on Eastern religion. Baer taught himself yoga and meditation. By the age of fifteen, he began his journey into the New Age world. Later he started experimenting with marijuana. He was certain the drug would expand his mind into what he called "higher consciousness."

In college, Baer became intrigued with American Indian culture, pantheistic religious views, and "getting back to nature." Encouraged by books written by Timothy Leary, Richard Albert (Ram Dass), and Aldous Huxley, he used hallucinogens and psychedelic drugs heavily.

As a religious studies major, Baer delved into Hinduism, Taoism, Buddhism, Yoga, and the teachings of Western mystics. He learned about such things as spirit guides, diagnosing health problems, dream control, techniques of mind over matter, psychic powers, and other thought power techniques for controlling reality. Well on his way into the New Age movement, Baer became involved with gurus and Transcendental Meditation where he received his own personal mantra.

After graduating with a B.A. degree in religious studies, Baer decided to pursue a course in holistic medicine. His first step was to attend a holistic health retreat in the San Juan Islands of Washington state. There he was introduced to a variety of techniques, including those that purport to realign the body's energy field. He went on a vision quest through a survival school in Provo, Utah. There, through a long period of meditation, he had a definite mystical experience. There, too, he was taught how to acquire a power helper for himself. He was a spirit hawk.

After two years, Baer graduated from a holistic health center with an N.D. (Naturopathic Doctor) degree. Many of his fellow students were nurses and former nurses who were disillusioned with orthodox medicine. This worked out well, because the training was radically opposed to much of what orthodox medicine had to offer. Baer was taught such subjects as iridology, body/mind integration techniques, trigger point therapy, martial arts, spiritual awareness, and herbology.

From his insider's view as a practitioner in New Age medicine, Baer tells us, "The area of holistic health is one of the most subtle and sophisticated areas of the murky merging of the esoteric and the mundane, the metaphysical with the mainstream, the pseudo-scientific with the scientific, the non-New Age with the New Age."[6]

Later Baer met Vicky, the woman who has become his wife. Vicky had received a small, perfect quartz crystal from an American Indian medicine man. One of her spirit guides instructed her to give Baer the crystal and ask him to meditate upon it. At first Baer thought this was ridiculous. But his meditation convinced him that the crystal really did have power. Thus began his journey into the world of crystal healing.

Baer and his wife became more and more deeply involved in meditation and in contact with the spirit world. He talked with spirits who identified themselves as Mozart, Moses, White Eagle, White Cloud, Ascended Master Kuthumi, Mary, and a host of others. To him the power emanating from these spirits was overwhelming and utterly intoxicating.

If you need proof of New Age healing's involvement in the mainstream of life, take a look at the professional activities in which Baer was involved. He taught hatha yoga classes at the local YMCA. He taught "dynamic relaxation" classes through the continuing education branch of the state university. He gave lectures at the public library on "quartz crystals and self-transformation." He conducted crystal healing sessions at a popular local metaphysical book store. He taught aerobic classes at the YMCA. He was a staff member of a local holistic health school. He gave natural health care lectures to the general public. He coordinated a city-wide "New Age networking guide to Santa Fe." He organized a "New Age festival of light." He participated in various New Age conferences and expos in Santa Fe, and, on the side, he sold crystals at flea markets.

For a living, Baer and his wife ran a center in New Mexico where they worked in the areas of group channeling, acupuncture, past life incarnation, past life regression, UFO contact sessions, guided imagery for success and prosperity, stress management, and many other topics.

About three months after Baer moved to northern New Mexico, his spirit guides gave him instructions to write a book on the subject of crystals. Since it had only been one year since his first introduction to crystals, he had no idea how to accomplish this task, yet he set about it at once. Supposedly during various trance states, the spirit guides gave him explicit instructions concerning what he was to write and how he was to do it. "The spirit guides were transmitting their thoughts and influences to me," Baer recalls. "My job effectively was to take notes, then to shape up the material into book form."[7] He also says that a person in such a trance state is "highly vulernable" to demonic influence.

The spirit-channeled book, *Windows of Light: Quartz Crystals and Self Transformation,* released in 1984—just at a time when the idea of crystals was really taking hold—launched Baer into the national New Age scene.

During his fifteen years of experiences, Baer says he had the opportunity to see the wide variety of people who are drawn to the New Age movement—M.D.s, Ph.D.s, dentists, chiropractors, teachers, and other highly educated professional people. "It's incredible," he says, "the number of these people who would reveal to me that they found out they had been Moses, or Cleopatra, or Renoir, or Thomas Edison, or Michelangelo in their past lives. They had been in telepathic contact with UFO aliens, some would say, and they were going to be beamed up to some spaceship shortly."[8]

One evening when Bear was in a trance state, he had an experience that was to change his life forever. He was surrounded by overwhelming luminosity as if he were looking straight into the sun.

"Rays of bliss radiated through my spirit. I was totally captivated by the power," Baer writes. "Suddenly another force stepped in. It took me by complete surprise. In the twinkling of an eye, it was like a supernatural hand had taken me behind the scenes of the experience I was having. I was taken behind the outer covering of the dazzling luminosity and there saw something that left me literally shaking for a full week. What I saw was the face of devouring darkness. Behind the glittering outer facade of beauty lay a massively powerful, wildly churning face of absolute hatred and unspeakable abominations, the face of demons filled with the power of Satan."[9]

From Darkness to Light

According to Baer, the same supernatural hand delivered him from the jaws of this consuming darkness. Hours later, when he awakened, all he knew was that some force greater than the devouring darkness had done two things: It had shown him the real face of the New Age heavens and angels, and it had delivered him from certain doom. Only later did he discover that this saving power was that of Jesus Christ.

Romans 8:38–39 was to become vital to Baer. There the apostle Paul wrote that "neither death nor life, nor angels nor principalities nor powers, nor things present nor things to come, nor height nor depth, nor any other created thing, shall be able to separate us from the love of God which is in Christ Jesus our Lord."

When Baer became a Christian, he began to realize that many of the practices in which he was involved were wrong. He now says, that regardless of whether sacred science "works" to some degree or not, it is based on occult principles and practices that are forbidden in Scripture (see Deut. 18:9–12). We agree with Baer. This is the ultimate flaw of New Age sacred science.

Even so, Baer at first saw no inherent contradiction in being a Christian involved in crystals—to relieve stress, quiet headaches, or build up vitality—and the so-called New Age sacred science so long as he did not specifically involve himself in the forbidden practices listed in Deuteronomy 18:9–12: divination, astrology, sorcery, witchcraft, necromancy, consulting with familiar spirits, and wizardry. Crystals, Baer reasoned, were neutral unless they were used to tell fortunes or to call up spirit guides. He was soon to find out how wrong he was. He finally reached the conclusion that just because something works doesn't mean that it's true, and that Satan and his hosts can perform counterfeit miracles (see 2 Thess. 2:9).

If crystals do work, Baer now believes, not enough research has been done to enable us to control their power. This alone should prevent us from calling upon them. But there is an even more important consideration. The so-called sacred science of the New Age, and crystals, and all they encompass are nothing but an attempt at modern day sorcery, white magic, and wizardry, all of which the Bible specifically forbids.

Ultimately the Holy Spirit brought Baer to this understanding. Once he saw it, he renounced all involvement in the field of sacred science and crystals.

FLOWER REMEDIES

Meet Dr. Edward Bach, a homeopathic physician who developed the concept of flower preparations. Actually, it's not too surprising an idea if you accept the belief that there is some power in all natural substances.

"Flower essence" is a general term for a liquid preparation created by immersing a flower into water and exposing the preparation to sunlight or heat. According to the *Encyclopedia of Alternative Health Care,* this "infuses the preparation with healing properties that come from the life energies and spiritual elements contained in the flower."

Actually, Bach's idea isn't all that new. Here is yet another rework of the old energy theory that somehow or another we can get life energy from a natural substance and transfer it into a healing potion.

Bach, who believed that illness was a symptom of mental or emotional imbalance, turned away from drug treatments. Instead, he chose to explore the healing powers of nature. Picture it: Dr. Bach, roaming the countryside of Wales, examining all the herbs and plants he found during his morning walk. It was his practice to pause to sip the morning dew from particular flowers. Eventually he developed thirty-eight different flower remedies for specific emotional imbalances.

Bach believed that the unique healing power of a plant is in its energetic property, and that this can reestablish the link between body and soul, nature and spirit. He also practiced the muscle testing technique of kinesiology. He would have his patient hold a bottle containing the preparation to be tested, then he would ask either silently or aloud if the flower was appropriate for the problem. Gently he would test the resistance of the patient's outstretched arm.

Although flower remedies sound harmless enough, the basis is the same as that of all other energy manipulating practices.

From Flowers to Spirits

If you wish to see the extreme end of the spectrum of the alternative health care movement, consider the book written by "Gurudas," the spirit channeled by Kevin Ryerson, Shirley MacLaine's psychic. Spirit Gurudas lists in concise charts the flower essences he claims most useful to address specific diseases, organs, emotional problems, and professions.

Now, I can see no physical harm in using liquid preparations which are nothing more than flowers dipped in water. A person would get no more than flower scented water. It's the other aspects of the procedures that cause me concern.

One flower therapist says, "I tell my clients to hold drops under their tongues while opening themselves to the healing vibrations of the flowers. Then I ask them to say an affirmation, get a picture in their mind of a wanted outcome, or just think about why they are taking the essences."[10] What a wonderful chance for anyone using flower essence to create her own reality. This very point is at the heart of most, if not all, the alternative health care practices.

IRIDOLOGY

Just when you think you've heard everything, something more ridiculous comes along.

Margaret, one of the nurses discussing therapeutic touch with me over lunch, had been to a workshop on iridology, a "science" in which the iris of the eye is consulted for diagnosis and treatment. "It's like what a physician does. He looks into his patients' eyes all the time to see what's wrong."

You can believe I took offense. To consider a physician's examination of the retina with iridology is not only ridiculous; it's an insult to the scientific practice of medicine.

Window to the Body?

An advertisement for iridology states: "The physical condition of every area of our bodies is shown in our eyes as well as the mental and emotional state of every individual." As if this all-encompassing statement isn't enough, the ad continues: "This information is 100% accurate, for the eyes and our bodies are incapable of expressing anything other than what is true."

This makes no sense at all—Red Flag No. 8.

The iridologist who runs this ad—who, by the way, works out of a hair salon—says that "by using the science of iridology, an iridologist can determine any weakness or malfunction within our body." *Any* weakness or malfunction? Clearly we are into superlatives here.[11]

She goes on to say that a potential problem can show up in the eyes up to two years before actually manifesting itself as a physical condition. By reading your eyes, she claims, she can offer suggestions as to how you may bring about healing through natural means without the use of drugs or medication, before you even know you have anything that needs to be healed. Quite a feat, I'd say.

Like reflexologists, iridologists also use maps—eye charts that show parts and qualities of the eye that supposedly reveal information about the body's condition. No one seems bothered by the fact that numerous eye maps are available, many of which are not at all similar.

Iridologists claim that the iris is but an extension of the brain. Never mind that the iris isn't even nerve tissue, as are both the brain and the nervous system. Physiologically, there is no possible way the iris can do what iridologists claim it does.

100 Percent Effective

There is absolutely no way to achieve 100 percent accuracy in any medical diagnosis or healing method (Red Flag No. 6). No physician I know of would dare to claim to be perfectly accurate in even the simplest of diagnoses, much less to base such a claim on something as physiologically unsound as iridology.

Nevertheless, many scientific studies have been done to test the persistent claims of iridologists. An investigation in 1979 at the University of California at San Diego indicated clearly that iridology had absolutely no valid claim. The results of this scientific study were published in the *Journal of the American Medical Association,* September 28, 1979. Three world renowned iridologists gave their best effort to provide accurate diagnoses. All three failed miserably. Another study conducted at the University of Melbourne in 1981 reached the same conclusion: There are no detectable iris changes associated with the diseases indicated on the iridology eye charts.

Chiropractor Bernard Jensen, one of the more vocal proponents of iridology, has undeniably been influenced by the Hindu teachers of India, especially by Sai Baba, a guru whose claim to fame is that he can materialize grey ashes out of thin air. Baba's followers believe him to be the incarnation of many Hindu deities, as well as of Jesus Christ Himself. At the bottom of the back cover of Jensen's textbook on iridology is the Hindu symbol for the meditational word *om*.

Says Jensen:

> The science of iridology has shown that nearly everyone has inherent weaknesses in the body, and it is in these areas that toxins tend to settle, creating conditions that favor eventual breakdown from infection, disease, or some other malfunction.[12]

And just what does Jensen believe is the cure for these toxins? Enemas, he says, and colonic therapy.

Eye Maps

Jensen's text and other materials form a standard for the teaching of this so-called science. The way his eye map is set up is almost funny. The pupil of the eye supposedly corresponds to the navel, and the organs occupy areas in the iris in relation to their position to the navel. So we're supposed to believe that not only is there a correlation between the eye and other distant and unconnected organs, but that there is also a connection between the eye and the navel.

If any correct diagnoses ever come from this most unscientific of methods, then surely it is either blind chance or the result of the psychic or occult abilities of the iridologist.

One of the biggest dangers of iridology is delay. Real disease requires real treatment. Sometimes it requires *immediate* real treatment. Unscientific practices which postpone that treatment can prove deadly.

REFLEXOLOGY

An elderly aunt of David's lives in a small town in rural Texas. "I used to have headaches," she told us, "but not any more. A young woman comes in to rub my feet, and now my headaches are much better."

The young woman is a reflexologist. As she sits with our aunt, rubbing her feet, she listens to her, talks to her, and visits with her. It is the bright spot of our aunt's day.

Reflexology, also called zone therapy or compression massage, is another energy-manipulating practice commonly used in alternative health circles. This technique involves massaging a patient's feet at specific points in order to bring relaxation, pain relief, or some other physiologic change to a distant part of the body.

According to the *Encyclopedia of Alternative Health Care,* reflexology is merely an American refinement of oriental wisdom and practice. Although we most commonly think of foot reflexology, there is also hand reflexology, ear reflexology, zone therapy, and even body reflexology.

The originator of this treatment in America was an ear, nose, and throat specialist by the name of Dr. William Fitzgerald who introduced zone therapy in 1913. Heavily influenced by traditional Chinese medicine, Dr. Fitzgerald taught that the body's bio-electrical energy flows through zones to relax points in the feet and hands. Although his theory differed from the Chinese, both theories based their techniques on the principle of a life force that can be manipulated and enhanced through touch.

Eunice D. Ingham refined Fitzgerald's ideas and concentrated on the feet. Thus, in the 1940s began the teaching of foot reflexology, which still exists today.

Reflexologists not only believe their foot massages bring about physiological changes, they claim potential psycho-emotional benefits as well. Like the acupuncturists, zone therapists and reflexologists say that by massaging certain points on the body, blockages of universal life energy are released to flow freely through the body. Reflexology is especially attractive because it can be done so simply and requires virtually no training. Practitioners simply refer to a map of the foot to locate the area to stimulate for a particular purpose.

Literature published by the International Institute of Reflexology in St. Petersburg, Florida, says that reflexology is a science that works from the principle that reflexes in the feet relate to every organ and all parts of the body. (At this point we must question this definition of "science." It can't possibly be the same definition we use.)

The literature goes on to say that the original method of reflexology is primarily used for relaxing tension, and that it improves the blood supply and helps nature to normalize the body. Apparently in an effort to impress us with the healing abilities of reflexology, the *Encyclopedia of Alternative Health Care* says that although there are few reasons not to use reflexology, there are some cautions: "Stimulating circulation or energy may accelerate the spread of infection and other conditions compromised by increased circulation." That would be the least of my worries since, in general, improved circulation aids in fighting infection. (Red Flag No. 8 on not making sense is flying high once again.)

In an effort to prove the validity of reflexology, Dr. Ronald

Hoffman, medical director of a place called the Whole Life Medical Center of Manhattan, uses a line that is popular with the alternative health movement to explain why there is no scientific proof of this method. He says that reflexology has scientific validity that hasn't been discovered yet. He says it's an empirical science, but its validity has only been reported from the clinic, not the laboratory. (Primary proof from testimonies? Red Flag No. 10!)

So why does reflexology work? If it does seem to work, it's for the same reason many other alternative therapies seem to work: the placebo effect. David's aunt doesn't care why it works. She doesn't require scientific proof. She's getting what she paid for—someone to care about her. Let's hope she never suffers from anything more than a minor headache.

REIKI

In the *Encyclopedia of Alternative Health Care,* author Kristin Olsen says Reiki is "an energy healing system based on ancient Tibetan knowledge discovered by a Japanese theologian." Many people have commented on the ecumenical aspect of Reiki. Supposedly it was founded by Dr. Mikao Usui, a Japanese Christian minister in Kyoto, Japan, in the mid-1800s. When one of his students challenged his belief that Jesus Christ healed people with His hands, Dr. Usui began a quest for proof that this type of healing actually did exist.

Unable to find the answers he sought in the Bible, Usui learned the ancient language of Sanskrit and began to read the sutras, the ancient books of esoteric Hindu religious teaching. After years of study and meditation, he came upon what he thought was a healing knowledge he termed "Reiki." The name comes from the Japanese words *rei,* meaning "boundless and universal," and *ki,* meaning "vital life energy force that flows through all living beings."

The story goes that after discovering this healing in the sutras, Usui undertook a twenty-one day fast atop a mountain in Japan. On the final day of his meditative quest, he reported that a ball of light containing the symbols of what later would become Reiki hit him on the forehead. This new power proved itself to Usui when he stubbed his toe as he came down the mountain after the fast. His toe, he claimed, was immediately healed with his new energy healing system.

Reiki today is an energy technique that is passed along from Reiki masters to initiates. According to Olsen, these Reiki masters themselves don't understand how it works. They can only describe it as a linking with the cosmic radiant energy, an opening of chakras, or an attunement with universal life energy.

Olsen is struck by the similarities between the empowerment rituals of Tibetan Buddhism and the Reiki initiation ceremony. She describes it as a modern secular adaptation of ancient sacred knowledge used in healing and self-healing.

How Does It Work?

Reiki treatments consist of a series of three or four sessions lasting about an hour each. The practitioner's hands are held at twelve basic positions, for five minutes each. Although there are many possible hand positions, a practitioner allows his or her own intuition to guide the placing. Over problem areas, the holding time is doubled. During a Reiki session, the practitioner supposedly draws energy and focuses it through his hands, thus providing a link between himself and the patient. Some Reiki teachers have described this connection as "lighting up."

The technique, proponents say, can be applied to the practitioner himself, to other people, to plants, or to animals. Reiki practitioners say they can even heal long distance! They do not claim to diagnose or to possess medical skills. But with practice, they say they can detect energy responses from the body that often give clues to the site of an organic problem and its seriousness.

Is It Religious?

Reiki practitioners staunchly deny that what they do has anything to do with religion or God. The Reiki master is not a guru, they insist. However, one cannot fail to notice the channeling of universal energy which is the very basis of the Hindu prana and other energy manipulating techniques. No spiritual aspects? Indeed there are.

As in so many other techniques we have considered, evidence of Reiki healing relies on stories and testimonies. Often these are full of unexpected effects and cures, like the woman who taped her hand to her abdomen each night for weeks to relieve her abdominal cramps. Eventually her pain subsided, but first a wart fell off. Why? Supposedly because Reiki energy had its own healing agenda.

As with so many other questionable practices, Reiki is couched in medical disclaimers. A Reiki teacher named Michael O'Leary is quoted in the *Encyclopedia of Alternative Health Care* as saying this energy work can help the terminally ill, but "not so much to cure the cancer, because sometimes there is just not enough wholeness to expand to sustain physical life." Are you willing to stake your life on this kind of questionable therapy?

THERAPEUTIC TOUCH

Not long ago I had lunch with three nurses from the University of Texas Nursing School, a large institution here in Austin. Sue and Jeanne were in their late thirties, Margaret was around fifty. All three had Ph.D. degrees.

Sue had been heavily influenced by a trip she took to China. "Acupuncture," she said with obvious enthusiasm, "is a combination of both medical systems—Chinese and modern."

She went on to say that although nurses would never be allowed to practice acupuncture, she felt they could legitimately practice the technique of acupressure for minor aches and cramps. "I even used it once to revive someone who had fainted," she told us.

"Nursing gives us the right to touch people," Sue continued. "Not all professions have that right."

Sometimes, Sue admitted, she practiced what she called "sneaky acupressure." That is, she performed it without the patient's knowledge.

"I can't go along with all of acupuncture," Sue told us, "but I believe it works because of the energy." That no one was able to detect this energy really didn't bother her. "The reason we can't measure it is because we don't know enough yet."

With obvious sincerity she informed us, "I can feel an energy pulse which allows me to gauge my treatments. It's something like electricity, but it's not really the same." Then, in case we might doubt it, she emphasized, "It is totally real, though."

All three nurses were pleased to see that reflexology was "at last" coming into nursing texts. They informed me that there was a program in Santa Cruz, California, set up by nurses, which instructs public school teachers in ways they can use acupressure on children with handicaps.

Although Sue said she couldn't diagnose what was wrong with a patient by "reading the energy field," she insisted she could tell if the energy field was distorted when the patient was sick, because unexplained energy pulsations could be found over any diseased areas.

"I channel energy from the universe down through my arm like a little flashlight," Sue said. "This takes practice, but you could learn to do it."

"We are simply looking for another way to help people," Margaret added.

Jeanne agreed. "We've given them medicine, we've given an I-V, we've cleaned them, we've turned them ten times, yet they are still in terrible pain. We can't just walk away. We've got to try something—anything that might possibly help."

In an honest attempt to help their patients, these earnest health professionals have begun to cross the boundaries of good sense. With spiritual naivete, they are tumbling headlong into the arena of the occult.

Healing Hands?

America's answer to Reiki is therapeutic touch. This technique was popularized by several registered nurses, including its founder, Dolores Krieger, Ph.D., who was also a professor at New York University. Dr. Krieger believes that anyone can be taught to sensitize himself to the "unnamed and unmeasured energy." As in Reiki, she insists that in therapeutic touch no religious faith is required, not by the patient and not by the practitioner.

Therapeutic touch is a laying-on-of-hands healing technique created for health care professionals to enhance the care and treatment of their patients. Although it was supposedly inspired by the effectiveness of psychic healing, it's designed to be done by non-psychics, those who simply want to help or heal.

A New York research team, made up of a physician and a self-proclaimed clairvoyant and healer named Dora Kuntz, was studying the effects of the direct laying-on-of-hands treatment of Oscar Estebany, a well-known Hungarian healer. Krieger joined the team and chose a biochemical measure for healer-energy influence, that of blood hemoglobin levels in the studies of nineteen medically referred subjects. The three researchers felt that hemoglobin, which is integral to the body's functioning, would be affected by such a healing energy.

So impressed was Krieger by the results of the studies involving this psychic that she decided to see if a non-psychic such as herself with no natural "healing ability" could learn to do what Estabany did in the experiment. Krieger claims she not only discovered how to feel the energy flow, but she learned to channel it as well.

In 1975, Krieger began teaching therapeutic touch, and, in 1979, wrote *The Therapeutic Touch: How to Use Your Hands to Help and Heal*. Therapeutic touch is still taught in a number of nursing schools throughout the country. In fact, it has become an international movement among the nursing profession.

Eastern Influence

It is Krieger's contention that the use of hands as a healing instrument is a gift we have forgotten in our scientific, mechanistic world. By her own admission, she has been heavily influenced by the health practices of yoga, ayurveda, and Tibetan and Chinese medicine. Also, she connects the Hindu and Yoga concept of prana to the rise in blood levels of hemoglobin in her research. Healers and healthy people, she believes, have an abundance of this prana, whereas the sick have a deficiency. And, still, she claims no Eastern religious involvement.

To her, therapeutic touch is like attaching jumper cables between a healer's charged battery and a sick person's low battery. The sick borrows energy from the well to jump start his immune system, and thus becomes better able to ward off the disease that afflicts him.

Author and registered nurse Janet Macrae says it this way:

> In a state of health, the life energy flows freely in, through, and out of the organism in a balanced manner, nourishing all the organs of the body. In disease, the flow of energy is obstructed, disordered, and/or depleted. Therapeutic touch practitioners, having learned to tune to Universal Field through conscious intent, direct the life energy into the patients to enhance their vitality."[13]

In therapeutic touch, the healer or nurse will "center herself in a meditative state." This focusing of her intent to help her heal the patient is a crucial step. According to studies on therapeutic touch, nurses who "did not center themselves or focus healing intent, but concentrated on counting backward in increments of seven, while going through the hand motions of therapeutic touch, showed no significant effects on their patients." The meditative state and focused intent, which we can now recognize as an altered state of consciousness, are vital components of therapeutic touch. (Healing energy and altered state of consciousness? Two red flags for therapeutic touch.)

Without a doubt, therapeutic touch has gained an amazing degree of respectability in medical quarters. New York University actually accepts it as a part of its master's curriculum in nursing. Because a Ph.D. nurse, Krieger, promotes its use, the technique has gained an aura of validity. In fact, a term occurring with increasing frequency in nursing conferences is that of so-called meta-nursing. Meta*physical* nursing would be a more accurate designation. Just consider the implications for the medical community!

The fact is, as Bob Larson points out, "Belief in a non-physical energy responsible for health and healing (such as occurs in therapeutic touch, Reiki, and other such energy balancing techniques) is common among occult healers."[14]

Alterations in universal energy, say its proponents, are the basis for all events which have previously been called supernatural or miraculous. Universal energy, they insist, is what religions through the ages have called God. But is it from God? You be the judge.

Never mind the "Force." May the one true God be with you.

Chapter Eight

COMMUNICATING WITH THE SPIRITS

Supernatural Therapies

"**I**'d like my boy here to have a physical examination," an attractive young woman named Beth said to me. "And while you're at it, why not check him for anemia and hypoglycemia?"

"Why those conditions?" I asked. "Does he have any symptoms?"

"No," Beth answered, "but a psychic told me I should have him checked."

When I asked why she went to the psychic, she said she wanted to learn more about her parents who had died in an automobile accident when she was a child.

"My mother used to consult psychics," Beth told me.

For the $60 she paid for the half-hour reading, Beth was assured her parents were fine, but the psychic went on to tell her that her children needed blood tests.

The woman, Beth said, could extract information from people she couldn't possibly have known. Beth called this a "psychic reading." I call it a con game.

For hundred of years magical efforts to gain control over nature by means of secret words, incantations, ceremonies, and various concoctions have represented a sort of primitive technology. Many of today's holistic practices aren't all that different.

Anne Stein calls herself a healer, a psychic, a witch, and a priestess of the goddess craft. An educated woman with a master's degree in English literature, she offers us insights into witchcraft through her book *Stroking the Python*. The very first chapter deals with altered states of consciousness. It's an appropriate beginning. Altered states are key to many alternative healing methods, and always a major red flag.

CALLING IT "CHRISTIAN"

Dave Hunt, in *The Seduction of Christianity: Spiritual Discernment in the Last Days,* says visualization and guided imagery have long been recognized by sorcerers of all kinds as the most powerful and effective way of contacting the spirit world for the purpose of acquiring supernatural power, knowledge, and healing.

Hunt points out that Episcopalian priest and Jungian psychologist Morton Kelsey, through seductive reasoning, persuades the church to believe that witchcraft, sorcery, and other forms of shamans are not evil in themselves, but are legitimate so long as we use them lovingly and for good. Kelsey writes:

> When we look at the ministry of Jesus we shall see . . . that his life and acts, his teaching and practice, are rather akin to shamans based on an intimate relationship with the loving Father God. In fact, an important study might be made comparing the ministry of Jesus with that of shamans.[1]

Kelsey goes on to say that the shaman is the mediator between the individual and spiritual reality, both good and evil, and because of this is the healer of diseases of both mind and body. In stepping into His healing role, Jesus picks up the prophetic and shamanistic strand of the Old Testament tradition, according to Kelsey. (Red Flag No. 12: Christian endorsements are no guarantee of legitimacy!) That Jesus healed by virtue of His power and authority as the actual Son of God and not by magical incantations uttered in a shamanistic trance seems to have escaped Kelsey.

New Age proponents sometimes mix the occult with Christianity in books like *The Jesus Letters*, which is being sold through New Age catalogues and stores. Two Connecticut women, Jane Palzere and Anna Brown, claim that the book was communicated to Palzere in 1978 and 1979 through a process known as "inspirational writing." Many spiritists use this technique of automatic writing to contact the spirit world.

Palzere and Brown's communicating spirit identified himself as Jesus—the biblical Jesus of Nazareth, the authors insist. The spirit dictated a series of one-page letters on such contemporary concerns as the energy crisis, abortion, marijuana, divorce, adoption, and suicide.

To make it still more confusing, this book is endorsed by several respected authorities such as Dr. Norman Vincent Peale. Dr. Peale says, "What a wonderful gift to all of us is your book . . . You will bless many by this truly inspired work. The book is interesting. God does not see evil. He sees only souls at different levels of awareness."[2]

What Dr. Peale and others like him are overlooking is that the Old and New Testament contain numerous passages saying God does see and hate evil. It also contains passages with God's commands concerning communication with the dead or spirits. We have previously noted that God gave this last admonition to the children of Israel before they entered the Promised Land after wandering forty years in the wilderness:

> There shall not be found among you anyone who makes his son or his daughter pass through the fire, or one who practices witchcraft, or a soothsayer, or one who interprets omens, or a sorcerer, or one who conjures spells, or a medium, or a spiritist, or one who calls up the dead. For all who do these things are an abomination to the LORD. And because of these abominations the LORD your God drives them out from before you (Deut. 18:10–12).

Not much to question here. Clearly, these occult practices are prohibited in God's eyes. Yet within the realm of holistic healing and the New Age medicine movement, they abound. In some cases they are wholeheartedly embraced by both practitioners and participants. In other cases they are tolerated alongside the seemingly good aspects of the New Age movement.

The book *Healers on Healing,* a compendium of thoughts from leading New Age healers and practitioners, contains contributions from several modern day shamans. In fact, 16 percent of the contributing authors claim to be practicing shamans. A look at the *National New Age Yellow Pages* also reveals a great deal about the scope and depth of the occultic elements in the New Age movement. Along with the acupuncturists and herbalists and naturopaths are sections on such practitioners as astrologers, spirit channelers, crystal therapists, interpreters of dreams, psychic healers, and sellers of magic potions and supplies.

Occult practices strike close to home. To hear Joan Quigly tell it, she was the real force behind the White House during the Reagan days. As President Reagan's former astrologer, Quigly grandiosely asserts that her astrological calculations were responsible for the success of Reagan's cancer surgery in 1985. She also claims to have controlled the nomination of Supreme Court justices, the meeting times for superpower conferences, and travel plans regarding the president and the first lady.

Far and wide, institutions and organizations involved with holistic health claim a psychic and spiritual dimension beyond the realm of the natural. They can be found in your hometown and mine, all seeking the New Age health dollar, all looking for converts to their way of thinking.

HOW IS IT MEDICAL?

A particularly disturbing organization here in the Austin area is one called the Healing Alliance. According to its Spring 1989 catalogue, this organization is led by a channeler who channels a spirit by the name of "Isaiah." The organization offers channeling classes, has a staff psychic and a practicing astrologer. In the channeling classes, Isaiah says, "Ask to be a channel and you are. By far the most difficult thing for you to do is trust the truth that will come to you."

"Okay," you may say, "but things like channeling and astrology aren't really medicine."

You wouldn't think so, would you? But consider the American Holistic Medical Association. Founded in 1978, its purpose was to unite licensed physicians who practice holistic medicine. Membership is open to medical doctors, osteopathic physicians, and medical students studying for those degrees. The stated purpose of the organization is to educate both professionals and the public, to support holistic physicians, and to promote preventive and holistic health principles.

In March of 1990, this organization held its thirteenth annual scientific conference in Seattle. The conference title was "Healing Our Planet Together: Holistic Concepts Applied to Personal, Professional, and Global Health." Sounds like a noble goal. Among the many courses offered at the conference was "Native American Medicine for the Modern World." Here attendees learned the philosophical basis of Native American rituals and ceremonies, about herbs and foods, group healings, Native American medical concepts, and how to use them. It even included a sweat-lodge ceremony.

More and more, the supernatural is seeping into mainstream medicine. C. Norman Shealy, M.D., writes:

We have consistently turned to faith healing by shaman and medicine men, by Great Mother and priest, and the witch doctor has imperceptibly faded into today's doctor. The strange paint and bizarre clothing of the ancient witch doctor have turned into the white coat and the hospital green mask and cap and operating gown, plus rubber gloves, leaving only a tiny bit of skin and eyes visible (not so very different from the animal skins or feathers or paint of primitive people).[3]

Abandonment of science; the melting of occultic spiritual practices with modern healing; doctors, nurses, and others all clamoring for a return to primitive medical practices with a New Age spiritual orientation: It's time that patients and the medical community alike squelch this rising tide of modern shamanism.

CHANNELING

Don't worry about nuclear war—"The Soviet Union and the U.S. are capable of setting aside their conflicts and allowing adept researchers to come together to find solutions to these problems that will destroy your planet, long before nuclear warfare."

We're all working toward the same end—"Human beings want the same things: to express themselves freely with no fear."[4]

How do we know these things? Why, from a spirit named Mena. He is channeled by a young woman named Gayle Reynolds Stauffer. Channeling is the technique by which a person acts as the channel or conduit for spiritual information from some spirit entity.

Perhaps the most famous recent example of channeling is outlined in Shirley MacLaine's well publicized book, *Out on a Limb*. Shirley MacLaine's personal channeler, Kevin Ryerson, purports to show us that we can indeed communicate with the other world. And other-world beings apparently would like very much to communicate with us.

Channeling with its direct and open invitation to demonic influence seems fraught with potential harm, both physical and spiritual. For many in the alternative medicine movement, the lure of occult knowledge is simply too great to resist.

Lazaris and Company

In the June 1989 edition of *New Age Holistic Health* magazine *Body, Mind, Spirit,* contributing editors include contributions from Seth, a spirit channeled by Jean Loomis; and from Lazaris, a spirit channeled by Jack Purcell, a Los Angeles art dealer who previously earned his living selling insurance. Channelers practice in every major city and in many rural communities in our country. If you prefer, you can get a reading by phone or by mail—for a nominal fee, of course.

According to Bob Larson, in *Straight Answers on the New Age,* Jack Purcell has turned Lazaris into a money making machine. Larson says Purcell averages nearly $200,000 per public transcendental discourse. He has a two-year waiting list for private consultations to the tune of $93 per hour. Simply to reach out and touch Lazaris by phone will set you back $35 per half hour—but it can be billed to your MasterCard or VISA.

Sharon Gless, of television fame, consults Lazaris. She even thanked him from the podium when she won an Emmy award. "Lazaris," she declared, "it is magic!"

Lazaris has a lot to communicate on topics ranging from how to heal the wounds of Vietnam to an explanation of how crystals were used in early civilizations such as Atlantis and Egypt. He also tells of other spirit guides—he calls them "unseen friends"—that surround humanity.

In various cities across our country are Seth Societies which study the teachings of Seth, the spirit guide of the late Jane Roberts. Seth preached a clear sermon of reincarnation: "There is not just one dimension in which non-physical consciousness resides. You must die many times before you enter this particular plane of existence. There is no need to fear death."

According to Bob Larson, J. Z. Knight is one of the best-known channelers. Knight channels the 35,000 year old spirit guide Ramtha. She claims Ramtha came to her in her kitchen while she was experimenting with crystal pyramids. According to Russell Chandler, author of *Understanding the New Age* and religion writer for the *Los Angeles Times,* channelers are yesterday's seance medium, palm reader, crystal ball gazer, and fortune-teller—dressed up in high tech drag and packaged by Madison Avenue.

Channelers run the gamut from Kevin Ryerson, who claims to channel such entities as John, a middle-East scholar from Jesus' day; to Tom McPherson, an Irish pickpocket who served the English diplomatic corps during the Shakespearean era; to a Brazilian channeler named Gaspareto, who runs a "spiritist center" for the poor in Sao Paulo and airs a weekly psychic television show. Gaspareto claims to channel about fifty "old master" artists, including Renoir, Picasso, Goya, and Toulouse-Lautrec.

The next time you're at Sea World or your local planetarium, think about Rev. Neville Rowe, a graduate electrical engineer, who says he channels dolphins as well as Soli, an off-planet being from the Pleiades star system. (Come on, Neville—a psychic link with Flipper and E.T.?)

Channeled entities all seem to bring the same basic messages: Death is unreal; all is one; we are all divine beings who have chosen to exist as physical humans; in this life there are no victims, only opportunities; we can control reality through the powers of universal mind.

Should we accept at face value the mystical babblings of these unseen spirits? We do so at our peril. Occultic consultation can be addictive, eventually controlling large portions of our lives and seductively indoctrinating us with distorted ideas of spirituality.

Emerging Acceptability

Mediums have been an integral part of nature religions almost since the dawn of time. Until recently, because of the predominant Judeo-Christian influence, mediums generally kept their practice with the spirit world secret. The Old Testament, claimed as holy Scriptures by Jews, Moslems, and Christians alike, condemns those who "have a familiar spirit." God specifically forbade His people from consulting spirits (Deut. 18:10–12).

In the early 1800s, however, spiritualism suddenly began to attract many prominent people. Thomas Edison spent years trying to devise an electronic means of communicating with the spirits of the dead. Queen Victoria, who had the longest reign of any monarch in British history, routinely consulted mediums. The presence of an astrologer in the White House should come as no surprise to students of history; seances were regularly conducted in the White House during Abraham Lincoln's presidency. Both Lincoln and his wife believed in spirits and in communication with the dead, and even made a number of attempts to contact their two dead sons.

It was psychologist Carl Jung who restored respectability to spiritism by suggesting that mediums were actually contacting deeper levels of their own psyches or the collective unconscious. Based on his recommendation, many psychologists have been at the forefront of this modern revival.

In the 1980s, mediumship took on a new name: channeling. Although there are certainly examples of frauds claiming to be mediums for financial gain, the evidence seems to support the distinct probability that spiritual entities really do exist and that they are the explanation of true mediumship and channeling. Although many scientists find the possibility of another dimension—a spiritual world—hard to believe, most of the major religions of the world readily embrace the concept of a "spiritual" dimension.

Today's spirit channelers act as if they have discovered something new. Yet we know that Old Testament biblical texts not only acknowledge spiritual beings but specifically counsel against involvement with mediums. Many of today's alternative practitioners do not heed this biblical warning, believing instead that only good can come from such spiritual contact.

New Age think tanks such as the Institute of Neotic Sciences readily affirm the existence of spirit beings. The institute's president likens the reluctance of today's scientific community to accept the existence of spirits to the French Academy of Science's attitude toward meteorites in the eighteenth century. Those who claimed to have seen flaming stones falling out of the sky were hallucinating, the academy insisted. It couldn't happen. There are no stones in the sky to fall.

No so very long ago, nobody ate tomatoes. No wonder. Every

American knew they were poisonous. Then someone proved that tomatoes weren't poison. Now everyone eats them.

Flaming stones do fall from the sky. Tomatoes are not poisonous. And spirits do exist. The apostle Paul wrote in his letter to the Ephesians: "For we do not wrestle against flesh and blood, but against principalities, against powers, against the rulers of the darkness of this age, against spiritual hosts of wickedness in the heavenly places" (Eph. 6:12).

Today's channelers seek power and knowledge from the spirits they consult. Unquestioning, they promote the spirits' message, perhaps never realizing the potential for deception from these demonic entities.

Jesus, the Ultimate Channel?

One famous "channeled" work is a book entitled *A Course in Miracles,* channeled by Helen Schucman, who at the time was a psychology professor at Columbia University and an avowed atheist. She claimed to be a medium for Jesus, who was supposed to have communicated the contents of the course to her. This three-volume course teaches only love. Sins have no effects at all; "they are but dreams." Guilt is impossible because the real self does nothing wrong. Forgiveness occurs when we realize there's nothing to forgive. There is no death, just a belief in death.

Amazingly, this course is taught in many churches throughout the country. It is the basis of the teaching for the Center For Attitudinal Healing, founded by California psychiatrist Gerald Jampolski, who himself was guided by his own "inner voice," or spirit, to a place where the principles of a course in miracles were demonstrated. (Red Flag No. 12 once again—Christian words are no guarantee of genuineness.)

Edgar Cayce

Is it possible for spirit guides to truly bring about healing? Assuming we accept the possibility that spirit entities exist, of course, it's possible. But there's a bigger question: What is the source of this power? Do spiritual entities represent a benign force of the universe, or are they perhaps disguised as "angel[s] of light" (2 Cor. 11:14).

Consider Edgar Cayce. For over forty years he diagnosed various causes of illness and prescribed therapy with a remarkable success rate that would be the envy of any physician. He simply fell asleep and entered a self-induced trance. The name and location of a patient was read to him, and without any indication of the symptoms, he announced in a firm voice, "Yes, we have the body." Then he launched into a reading, or an explanation of the cause of the illness, followed by a detailed prescription. This might include a special diet, medications—sometimes current and sometimes outdated—manipulation, massage, electricity, enemas, or homeopathic remedies.

The Cayce legacy lives in the Association for Research and Enlightenment (ARE), which has collected almost 9,000 of these medical "readings" from Cayce and letters from patients. It is the largest body of paranormal documentation related to healing.

Rolling Thunder, an American Indian medicine man, says that from what he has studied of the Cayce documents, Cayce's work fits nicely with American Indian prophetic healing.

Other testimonials to Cayce include one from Norman Shealy, M.D. and Ph.D., first president of the American Holistic Medical Association. Says Shealy, "My first visit to ARE in 1972 marked the beginning of my own transformation towards holistic health. I return each year to nurture myself among friends as one of the truly inspirational havens of the world."[5]

Edgar Cayce was born in Hopkinsville, Kentucky, in 1877. His grandfather was a water witcher. Both his grandparents could make tables and chairs move without touching them. As a child, Cayce claimed he was able to see "little people," or companions, in the fields.

The beginning of Cayce's diagnostic ministry was also the beginning of a lifetime of trouble with his voice. He had recurring voice failures, and was completely dependent upon his trance state to return his voice to normal. Once the physical readings had begun, Cayce could not abandon them. He had no control over whether or not they would occur, and if so, when they would come.

By the age of thirteen, Cayce had supposedly read through the Bible for the twelfth time. During his so-called readings, he often quoted Scripture. At one time he taught Sunday School in the Christian church, and he became a prominent leader in Alabama's Christian Endeavor organization. Yet about thirty percent of his life readings had to do with the lost continent of Atlantis, a secular and occult version of Noah's Ark.

Sometimes the treatments Cayce recommended seemed completely unrelated to the illness. When his wife, Gertrude, was reportedly dying of tuberculosis in 1911, he prescribed a trance-given regimen of liquid heroin capsules, interspersed with apple brandy fumes she inhaled from a charred keg. She survived.

Although he was investigated by numerous scientists and reporters, Cayce was never charged with fraud. In 1923, he traveled to Dayton, Ohio, to give an astrological reading to a wealthy Dayton printer. At the end of the horoscope, Cayce's trance-voice announced, "This printer once was a monk." Cayce had entered into a new world for him—reincarnation. Although he first rejected the whole idea of reincarnation, he later managed to reconcile his belief system with the readings he was doing.

Frequently Edgar Cayce questioned whether his work was of God or of the devil. The argument he used to quell his doubts was that if something good was accomplished, the work must be from God. Healing people's sick bodies was obviously good, and for thirteen years that was just what he had been doing. The voice within him had never lied. "It hasn't ever done evil and it won't let me do it," he said confidently.

Although Cayce may have felt comfortable with his unusual method of healing, the hallmarks of demonic possession were clear in his life, particularly in his trance states. Gary North notes that two of the criteria of demon possession used by the Roman Catholic church are: (1) the ability to gain access to information not otherwise obtainable by normal means; and (2) the ability to speak in foreign languages without prior instruction. Cayce's career exhibits both traits. Clearly, his healing methods and medical advice were unobtainable by normal means. And Cayce reportedly spoke in French, Italian, Spanish, German, and Tutonic German, as well as in several unknown tongues. A third criterion, a demonstration of superhuman strength, was never exhibited by Cayce.

Yet Cayce's philosophical and cosmological speculations indicate his trance states were indeed demonic. In an interview with the Dayton printer, Cayce said, "What you've been telling me today and what the readings have been saying is foreign to all I've believed and been taught, and all I have taught others all my life. If ever the devil was going to play a trick on me, this would be it."

After years of studying the Bible and trying to integrate biblical Christianity into his occult readings, Cayce finally succumbed to the persistent lure of the occult. If Christians have any doubt as to the identity of the Jesus to whom Edgar Cayce referred, they should note that he described Jesus as but one of some thirty incarnations of "the master." This spirit also appeared to Cayce as a variety of Old Testament notables such as Adam, Enoch, Joseph, and Joshua, and also as Hermes Trismegistos (the Egyptian god Thoth)!

According to Gary North, the Hindu concept of karma is at the heart of Cayce's movement. Karma is the ancient Eastern concept of the good or bad effects of the deeds done in this life. Every soul, to the extent that it is personal at all, lives numerous times working out the effects of karma. Sometimes they rise toward God, sometimes they fall away from God, but always they get another chance.

In many of Cayce's readings and in all of his books he quotes the biblical phrase, "You must reap what you sow." (The Bible states this as something that is to occur in the final judgment, not in numerous reincarnations.) Cayce believed "the master" (the reincarnated Jesus, Adam, Joshua, Hermes Trismegistos) took on human form at the time Atlantis was formed. In fact, he believed Atlantis was the biblical Eden.

"When did Jesus become aware he would be the saviour of the world?" Cayce would be asked.

His answer was always, "When he fell in Eden." Here the master began his series of incarnations, Cayce claimed. After becoming Enoch, then Joseph, then Joshua, then others, he finally became Jesus. The great master was supposedly incarnated a total of thirty times. Not only are Cayce's teachings unbiblical, stripping Jesus of any semblance of being God's Son, but he, like others who believe in reincarnation, was deluded by a grandiose reincarnated view of himself. Cayce believed that the channeled Thoth, a pyramid builder, had a partner who was a priest, Ra Ta—an early incarnation of none other than Cayce himself.

Prophets, True or False?

The Reverend Laura Camron-Fraser, from the Seattle area, the first woman Episcopalian priest in the Pacific Northwest, was forced to leave her church because she says a spirit named Jonah spoke through her. Arguing that trance channeling is how the Holy Spirit speaks to people today, she says, "We have to see the Bible as a channeled work. The prophets in the Old Testament were channelers."

Certainly the prophets were speaking the Word of God, but there was a stipulation applied to anyone who made such claims of prophecy. He had to be 100 percent accurate. No mistakes, no misquotes, no misunderstandings. For those who failed, the penalty was death (Deut. 18:20–22).

Were the same penalty demanded today, I wonder how many channelers would be speaking on Donahue, Merv Griffin, and prime time network television? Kevin Ryerson claims only 75 percent accuracy. I haven't found any other channeler willing event to suggest such reliability.

Texe Marrs, author of *Dark Secrets of the New Age,* identifies the consistent spiritual falsehoods that channelers put forward as: (1) a personal God does not exist, (2) Jesus is not the only begotten Son of God and is not the only Christ, (3) Jesus did not die for our sins, (4) there are no such things as sin and evil, (5) there is no Trinity of Father, Son and Holy Spirit, (6) the Bible is filled with errors, (7) there is no heaven and no hell, (8) every man is god and one's godhood can be realized through the attainment of a higher consciousness.

Can there be such a thing as a Christian channeler? Absolutely not!

PSYCHIC SURGERY

Meet Arigo, a Brazilian peasant who for over two decades, from 1950–1970, is said to have treated as many as 2 million patients. For almost twenty years, he spent six hours a day, five days a week, running over 300 patients a day through his "clinic." He would spend about one minute on each patient—including making a diagnosis, treating the person, and/or writing a prescription. Arigo was the king of psychic surgeons.

Like many other faith healers and miracle workers, as a boy Arigo was not a good student. In fact, he dropped out of school after third grade. From his earliest years he experienced flashes of eerie light and hallucinations. He said he heard a voice that spoke to him in a strange language. In time he was able to recognize the language as German.

Eventually the voice identified itself as the spirit of Dr. Adolpho Fritz, a German physician who died in 1918 and intended to use Arigo to complete his unfinished work. (It didn't explain why a Brazilian peasant was necessary to complete the work of a German physician.)

Arigo began to suffer severe headaches. Nothing could cure them, not even an official church exorcism. When Arigo finally consented to begin the work of Dr. Fritz, the headaches immediately ceased. They began again only once—when he temporarily discontinued the healings.

Apparently whatever power allowed him to heal had possessed Arigo. If he didn't heal, he couldn't avoid the headaches and the dreams. He was trapped.

Arigo's Fame Spreads

Arigo's healing ministry took a dramatic turn when Brazilian Senator Bittencourt came through Arigo's district. The senator had recently been told he was suffering from lung cancer, and he was returning to the United States for immediate surgery and treatment. Arigo spent the night in the same hotel as the senator. Sometime during the night Arigo, seemingly in a trance, reportedly entered the man's room carrying a razor. Bittencourt blacked out. When he awakened in the morning, his pajama top was slashed and blood was on both his chest and pajamas. There was a neat incision on his rib cage. The senator went to his physician, who x-rayed him and pronounced all traces of the cancer gone.

From this point on, Arigo's fame as a healer spread far and wide. Brazil was the perfect place for his talents, since numerous healing cults existed there, many of which involved spirits as well as other types of "alternative treatments." Spiritists were quick to claim Arigo for their own. In 1968 he openly stated, "All my family are Catholic. I am a spiritist, but I believe that all religions take people to God."

Under Arigo's powers, numerous healings occurred. A woman dying of cancer of the uterus was brought to Arigo. In front of her dazed family, he went into a trance, grabbed a knife, and thrust it into her body. He twisted and jabbed, making the opening wider and wider. Finally he reached into her womb and yanked out a tumor the size of a grapefruit. Arigo returned to the kitchen, dropped the knife and the tumor into the sink, then collapsed into a chair.

The physician who had diagnosed the woman's cancer was immediately called. The woman wasn't bleeding at all. She felt fine. The doctor took the tumor for examination. There was no possible medical explanation for the tumor's removal, the woman's survival, or the disappearance of all traces of her cancer.

Arigo wrote long, complicated medical prescriptions in a

matter of half a minute, often while staring blankly into space. Sometimes he prescribed long forgotten drugs. On other occasions the drugs were so new they were not yet available in Brazil. Strangely enough, the weird prescriptions, often given in abnormally high dosages, wouldn't work when any other physician tried them.

When Arigo was investigated for possible charges of practicing medicine without a license, not one person could be found to testify that he had injured anyone or defrauded anyone of money. Apparently, there was not one dissatisfied customer among the 2 million patients he had treated. Given the current number of lawsuits, this is a remarkable record indeed. Either Arigo was a colossally clever and successful fraud, or there was a supernatural force behind him.

Arigo's patients suffered no pain, little fear, little bleeding, and no scarring. On numerous occasions, his work, witnessed by physicians at close hand, was recorded on movie film and run and rerun in slow motion. Yet no one ever detected a single sign of fraud, manipulation, or sleight of hand.

In 1964, Arigo finally was convicted of practicing medicine without a license and was sent to jail, where he immediately started healing the prisoners. His imprisonment didn't last long. Despite such obstacles, patients continued to pour through Arigo's clinic.

Arigo had seen a black crucifix hanging in the air several times. One day in January of 1971, he bid a strange farewell to his friends. Just outside his hometown he was impaled in a violent auto accident and died.

To this day, researchers have failed to come up with an explanation of Arigo's abilities. In fact, his flagrant violation of basic fundamentals of cleanliness, anesthesia, and anatomy seemed calculated to insure that no explanation could possibly make sense other than that of Fritz's invisible skill.

Most Are Frauds

Arigo was a great exception among psychic surgeons. Most are out and out frauds who never do any real surgery at all. Yet

Kurt Koch, author of *The Occult ABC's,* states, "Let us be quite clear about this. Arigo's cures were not a trick or a swindle. They were real operations." Certainly they were not the work of God. Arigo was not possessed by a dead German doctor. He was possessed by a demon.

Because of Arigo, the tradition of spirit possession became even more firmly grounded in the minds of Brazilian peasants. Spiritists gained a new impetus—by 1960 some 680,000 were recorded in Brazil. The curse of real demonic healing, you see, is not that it doesn't work. The curse is that it might work. Accepting what their eyes see, desperate people willingly submit their bodies to the hands of demons to gain a few more years of life.

Yet psychic surgery is usually pure fakery, a fraud accomplished through sleight of hand, tricks, and devices. For every Arigo who truly heals, there are hundreds of fraudulent psychic surgeons. Nor are they confined to the jungles of Brazil. In fact, they can be found right here in Texas. Gary Cartright wrote an article in the *Texas Monthly* magazine's December 1986 issue entitled, "Touch Me, Feel Me, Heal Me." In it he told of a healer by the name of Angel Domingo, who showed up in the Austin area. Although there were no set fees for his services, there was a collection box for "love offerings" just inside the door of the treatment room. The suggested offering was $30. One member of his staff estimated that the daily take exceeded $5,000.

Gary Cartright reported that upon arriving at the room where he was to be healed he had to sign a disclaimer, saying that the treatment would be religious rather than medical, and that he understood the "minister" made no promises regarding the outcome.

Eventually author Cartright was able to get some of the tissue purportedly removed in these bloody operations. After analyzing it, local pathologists reported the material was definitely not human. Analyzed blood stains were found to be cow blood diluted with water.

Dr. Gary Magno, an Arizona surgeon known as "Reverend

Monsignor," was arrested in Phoenix in 1986 while "operating" in the home of one of his followers. He had been seeing a hundred patients a day, charging $75 for an initial visit and $50 for follow-up surgery. At the time of his arrest, Magno had vials of red fluid and packets of red meat tucked under his waistband.

In 1986, Jose "Brother Joe" Bugarin was said to have performed 360 surgeries in three days while sponsored by a Denver church. Although patients signed disclaimers, stating they were receiving "spiritual assistance," and although they knew Brother Joe was not licensed to practice any form of medicine, he was arrested after performing an "operation" on an investigator from the Colorado State Board of Medical Quality Assurance. Bugarin eventually served nine months in jail for practicing medicine without a license.

Unfortunately, the gullible include desperate parents who bring their children for treatment. Pediatric oncologist Ronald Chard, M.D., reported the cases of four children who had been treated by such fraudulent healers in the Philippines. All four died. In each case, Dr. Chard said, "I had the opportunity to observe the condition of the patients both before and after their treatment by the psychic surgeons. In each case, with the exception of one, the chances of the child having a longer life span would have been greater if conventional medical treatment had not been significantly interrupted."[6]

It's difficult to lump the spirit-possessed Arigo together with blatant frauds who use the pieces of dogs and cows and chickens to trick the public. What is clear is that psychic surgeons are either out and out frauds, or they are involved in the supernatural spirit world of demon possession and influence.

SHAMANISM

Anthropologist Michael Harner, an avowed shaman, defines a shaman as a man or woman who enters an altered state of consciousness at will to contact an ordinarily hidden reality for the purpose of acquiring knowledge and power. "Shamans," he writes, "who we in the civilized world have called medicine men and witch doctors, are the keepers of a remarkable body of ancient techniques that they use to maintain well-being and healing for themselves and members of their communities."[7] He goes on to say these shamanic methods are strikingly similar the world over, even in cultures that are quite different in other respects and have been separated by oceans and continents for tens of thousands of years.

Harner says the basic uniformity suggests that through trial and error various peoples arrived at the same conclusions. I have a different suggestion. Might it not be that there is a unifying force behind these practices? As we noted, Ephesians 6:12 affirms that the Christian warfare is against dark principalities and powers. The prince of this earth, Satan himself, may well be behind shamanic power.

The Essentials of Shamanism

There seem to be four essentials that are characteristics of a shaman's quest:

1. *A spirit guide.* In *The Way of the Shaman,* Michael Harner says that the shaman depends on special powers that are usually supplied by his guardian, and by other "helping spirits." Each shaman generally has at least one guardian spirit. Without this spirit, Harner says, it is virtually impossible to be a shaman.

These guides are believed to lead the shamans further and further into altered consciousness and to provide them with information on how to live their lives and heal others. It all comes from the spirit guide—which, according to Harner, should be trusted implicitly.

2. *An altered state of consciousness.* Healing, visions, advice, and knowledge from the other world supposedly occur only in an altered state of consciousness. The means for achieving this state are many and varied, including the repetitive drumming, frenzied sufi/dancing, and the repetitious droning

of a mantra: "Ohm, ohm, ohm." Transcendental Meditation has been at the forefront of promoting this altered state of consciousness.

Harner says that *some degree of altered state of consciousness is necessary for shamans to function*. In fact, he considers this the only way a spirit guide can be contacted.

3. *Astral travel.* This is what traditional shamans call the ecstatic journey. It is an out-of-body experience: The body remains where it is while the mind moves through cosmic planes of consciousness. In astral travel, the journeyer meets spirits and entities who may give them information, knowledge, and healing. The similarity between astral travel and near-death experiences (NDE) is perhaps more than coincidental.

4. *Influence from the spirit world.* The reason the shaman goes to the spirit world is to collect information and to gain knowledge not available to ordinary people. Does this mean shamans are possessed? If they are not controlled by these spirits, they are at least influenced by them. And they are compelled to believe and act upon anything these supernatural beings tell them.

Shamanistic Practice Vs. Medical Healing

Again, Michael Harner writes:

> The burgeoning field of holistic medicine shows a tremendous amount of experimentation involving the reinvention of many techniques long practiced in shamans such as visualization, altered state of consciousness, aspects of psychoanalysis, hypnotherapy, meditation, positive attitudes, stress reduction, and mental and emotional expression of personal will for help and healing. In a sense, shamanism is being reinvented in the West precisely because it's needed.[8]

But Harner assures us there is no conflict between shamanic practice and modern medical treatment. As an example, he points to the work of Dr. Carl Simonton and Stephanie

Matthews-Simonton in their treatment of cancer patients. Although the Simontons didn't knowingly pursue shamanic methods, Harner says, some of their techniques in support of cancer therapy are incredibly similar to those of shamans. For instance, they have patients relax in a quiet room and visualize themselves on a walking journey until they meet an inner guide which is a person or an animal. Then the patient asks the guide for help in getting well. Basically, this is nothing more than a shamanic journey, Harner says.

Harner envisions a day when modern shamanism can be practiced side by side with orthodox Western medicine. He hopes that all physicians will soon be trained in shamanic methods of healing and health maintenance, so both approaches can be combined.

Shamans have traditionally employed a wide variety of tools and techniques to connect themselves with the spirit world. One common technique is hallucinogenic drugs, such as peyote. Sometimes they also lay out power objects on a table or on the ground, each piece embodying the power it symbolizes.

One modern-day shaman and practicing physician is Dr. Louis Mehl. Dr. Mehl integrates his medical training with shamanic ritual, prayers, and stories from his Cherokee and Dakota background. A specialist in obstetrics, his medical practice includes visualization, somatic therapy, and biofeedback for women with high risk pregnancies.

Author Kristin Olsen, in the *Encyclopedia of Alternative Health Care,* recognizes that shamanism represents approaches and attitudes that are entirely different from the attitudes of the Judeo-Christian culture. Indeed it does! It is so different, in fact, that God has strictly forbidden His people to participate in it. Shamanism is an occultic practice.

Primitive Practice in a Scientific Age

For centuries the shaman was the only one in the primitive community who knew the connection to the spirit world. Today's holistic healers are encouraging the direct route. Any person, they say, can become his own shaman simply by seeking higher consciousness through meditation, guided visualization, and the pursuit of a spirit guide.

It's obvious why shamans appealed to primitive societies where little was known about the world. But what is their appeal to a society with advanced scientific knowledge? Americans understand vast realms not even imagined by ancient man. I believe the answer is simple: Our society has a spiritual void. The tragedy is that too many are trying desperately to fill this void through the deception of the occult.

C. S. Lewis said the two greatest dangers in considering the subject of Satan are, first, not to believe that demons exist; and second, to see a demon behind every bush. No, shamanism may not all be demonic—in many cases it may be pure fantasy. Yet we would do well to keep in mind that Satan's greatest deception is to get us to look inward rather than upward toward God.

Another attraction of shamanism is the idealized dream of a return to a simpler life. Many admire the American Indians of more than a century ago, with their close relationship to nature and their simple life-style. They didn't have to deal with technological contrivances such as CAT scanners and blood tests. They didn't worry about diseases such as AIDS and cancer. Of course, their life-span was considerably shorter than ours today and most of their daily efforts were directed toward issues of survival, such as finding food and shelter.

Many people are drawn into shamanism through their genuine concern with ecology and world peace. Only later are they confronted with the spiritual implications. We believe in ecology and peace too. Everybody should. But in the New Age movement, the tendency is to worship the creation rather than the Creator. Therein lies the problem. By using herbs and potions and the spirit world, many health care workers have become modern shamans, medicine men and spiritual authorities all rolled up into one.

VISUALIZATION

When Dr. Bernie Siegel made an appearance here in Austin, we went to see him. Several hundred people attended the meeting at an auditorium downtown. Dr. Siegel had been brought to town by a local New Age church and Sylvia Murray Productions, a group led by a self-proclaimed psychic and channeler.

The meeting began with a guided visualization led by Sylvia Murray. The crowd, mostly women, seemed familiar with the words she used: "consciousness," "at-onement," "meditate." In a hypnotic voice, Ms. Murray led the session in much the same way a Christian group begins a meeting with prayer.

We were told to "see a light within you." This light, she told us, was powerful, magical. "Let it fill you till you grow," she urged. "It heals everyone it touches." Her hypnotic voice went on: "We are healing the planet. Breathe deeply. Relax. Enjoy. You can live successfully, joyfully, like you want to. For as you see it, so shall it be."

When visualizing, a person conjures up an image of the idea or spirit he wishes to contact. Visualization may be enhanced by "centering," or focusing one's eyes on something such as a crystal, a mandella, or a candle flame. Sometimes the one doing the visualizing is encouraged to use a mantra to evoke his spirit guide.

Illusion or Reality?

Visualization has its roots in Hinduism, which teaches that all the universe is illusion. Only the spirit has substance. What we see around us and interpret as reality is really nothing but a figment of our imagination. If reality is an illusion, then mental powers can alter it. All we need do to make something different is to visualize it the way we want it to be. Hindus believe you can actually "create" your own reality, thus putting humans in the driver's seat instead of God.

This idea is especially appealing to the sick. Imagine being able to rid yourself of an illness simply by visualizing it away. Of course, they also believe if you aren't able to rid yourself of your disease, then perhaps you deserved it.

Visualization begins with relaxation techniques geared toward achieving an altered state of consciousness. The desired image is brought into the center of the mind, then is reinforced by repeated affirmations. This reinforcement may come in the repetition of a mantra, or perhaps in a particular thought: "I see myself well," or "I see my disease crumbling away." Negative or contradictory thoughts must be completely eliminated from the mind.

We're not talking positive thinking here. Visualization goes far beyond that. We're talking about creating a whole new reality.

In his book on healing visualization, Gerald Epstein, M.D., describes his imagery exercises as a "form of waking dreams— dreams that can make reality." He maintains that the medical and scientific world is highly interested in his techniques of visualization. However, at the beginning of his book Dr. Epstein, who is apparently well advised on the risks of medical malpractice, added a medical disclaimer. In discreet, fine print he writes, "This book is not intended as a substitute for medical advice of physicians. The reader should regularly consult a physician in matters relating to his or her health and particularly in respect to any symptoms that may require diagnosis or medical attention."[9] So much for his own confidence in this system of healing.

Who Knows Best, Doctor or You?

Just thirty-nine pages after that small print disclaimer, Dr. Epstein tells the story of Jennifer. After a gynecological condition that resulted in surgery, she was amazed to find she had guessed what was wrong with her before the doctors made their diagnosis. According to Dr. Epstein, Jennifer "knew more about herself than did her doctors." Not that Epstein was surprised. "Of course we know more about ourselves than anyone else can," he says. "All we need is the trust it takes to believe this. In Jennifer's case, one successful imagery experience was enough to encourage her belief and trust in herself."[10]

On the surface, this sounds fine. But if the physician is continually second guessed by a patient who allows her "intuition" to direct whether surgery should be performed, what medicine should be prescribed, and what diagnosis should be rendered, imagine the problems we'll encounter.

Dr. Epstein is no fool. He is well aware of the malpractice suits that can result from a doctor giving a patient wrong advice, either directly or in his books. So to be on the safe side, he gives another disclaimer, this one suggesting that the exercises in the book should not be used in place of prescribed medication or instead of seeing a doctor. This comes exactly one sentence after his statement that the imagery exercises in the following chapter are designed to help heal a large number of maladies, both physical and emotional. The long list includes AIDS, cancer, leukemia, bone fractures, multiple sclerosis, vaginal infections, acne, and thyroid disturbance.

To cure AIDS, for instance, he recommends imagery, meditation, prayer, diet, crystals, and healers. He then says, "In one documented case using Tibetan Buddhist meditation practice involving chanting and visualization, a woman succeeded in reversing the positive response of her antibody blood testing negative indicating all AIDS virus activity had ceased."[11]

As of now there is no known cure for AIDS. To suggest otherwise is criminal and negligent. If you were to demand proof from these people when they tried to pull the wool over your eyes, scientific evidence would seem to be the one thing that would not materialize.

Epstein also has some advice concerning inner guides, which he says sometimes appear when a person does imagery. He says you can achieve wonderful results without ever meeting a guide, but if you should encounter one while imaging you should not hesitate to take advantage of its services. In other words, blindly accept whatever this guide may say. Pay no mind to how it looks. Don't analyze what you are told. Disregard the nature of your relationship with this spirit guide. Just accept and obey. (Would you blindly accept anything else in your life without first evaluating it?)

Inner guides, says Epstein, come to people in whatever form

the specific person is best able to receive them, whether as animals, humans, or other-worldly creatures such as angels. Not only are we supposed to suspend skepticism, we're supposed to leave our minds parked at the door! We are to allow the spirit guide to take control, to tell us anything he wants, to manipulate our thoughts, to direct us down whatever paths he chooses to become puppets. This is contrary to the Word of God.

Magic. Witch doctors. Other-worldly spirits. Demon possession. These all play a major part in alternative healing. Many who have dabbled in the natural approaches, who have flirted with mind over matter, who have looked into universal energy, end up here in the supernatural.

Some will even swear by the fraud and fakery. We'll see why in chapter 9.

Chapter Nine

ANYTHING THAT WORKS IS OKAY

New Age Sugar Pills and Snake Oil

"It seemed like I was always getting sore throats," Jennifer told me. "My friend said I needed to clean out my system. So for two days I went on an all juice diet, mainly grape juice. It worked so well I now cleanse my system once a month. I don't get nearly as many sore throats anymore."

Hundreds of years ago medical practitioners were at a loss to explain why it was that a patient would get better or worse after a particular healing method was administered or withheld. We now understand a great deal more about sickness and health, but there is still a lot that mystifies us.

Why do certain treatments work?

Of course there are regimens and medications that have been tested and proven effective for certain conditions—antibiotics are a good example. As a physician, I deal with these treatments day in and day out. And there are undoubtedly many more therapies yet to come.

But what about those that have absolutely no basis in science? Patients extol the curative powers of homepathic remedies usually consisting of water or herbs, for example. Why do *they* sometimes seem to work?

There are several possible explanations. One is the natural course of events—the patient would have gotten well no matter what she did. This is true far more often than many patients realize. Many conditions are self-limiting; but if a patient is taking a certain preparation or following a particular course of treatment when she recovers, she is likely to credit it with her cure. If she was drinking grape juice, then the grape juice must have cured her. If she was soaking in warm baths, then the warm baths may have made her well.

Another possible answer is that the patient really did get better due to some specific feature of the treatment. When this is the case, the cure can be studied, isolated, or predicted by scientific medical means.

A third possibility is that the patient got better simply because she became more confident, had more hope and less anxiety. The cure was based at least partly on the psychological expectation of relief.

Doctors have long recognized that procedures which offer patients reassurance, whatever those procedures may be, can lead to marked improvement in that person's condition. This is "the placebo effect."

WHAT ABOUT PLACEBOS?

The word *placebo* is derived from the Latin meaning "I shall please." Sugar pills are a good example of this. As a young and somewhat immature medical student, I can remember seeing a woman in a hospital emergency room who had been brought in by her family because she suddenly couldn't walk. My physical examination revealed no obvious physical injury or disease and I was at a loss to explain her problem.

But the ER doctor had the answer, and a surprisingly simple solution. You see, he had seen this particular patient several times before, and each time his therapy was successful. This physician, who seemed extremely wise to me, produced a bottle of rather large pills marked OBECALP. I was not at all familiar with this medication. He gave one to the woman, who was amazingly calm in spite of the fact that she could no longer walk, and told her she would be well in ten minutes. Incredibly, about ten minutes later I saw this woman walk out the door.

A miracle cure? Magic? No, this woman had a recurrent psychological illness called a conversion reaction, and the doctor had given her some large sugar pills. The pills' strange name was PLACEBO spelled backwards.

Placebos have been given a bad name. Too often they are thought of as techniques for tricking patients into getting well. Yet the placebo effective is pervasive, and it has been credited with helping in such diverse maladies as coughs, mood changes, angina pectoris, headache, seasickness, anxiety, hypertension, asthma attacks, depression, the common cold, skin rashes, and all types of pain.

So what's the problem? If a person uses a placebo and actually gets well, and if he then stays well, what harm can it cause?

Sometimes, none at all. Other times, however, placebos lead patients straight into alternative medical techniques which, although they seem harmless on the surface, actually can be quite dangerous indeed.

In our society, people have come to expect quick, effective cures for everything that ails them. If they have any physical problems, they expect their doctors to "do something." And they want it done *now!*

There is great power in having a doctor prescribe a medication and assure her patient it will work. Honest physicians admit that the way in which a medication or treatment is given, and how the patient accepts it, has a good deal to do with how effective it will be. This can sometimes enhance the effectiveness of proven medical treatments. The holistic health movement, however, has readily embraced this idea.

Every physician has experienced the mother who brings her child to him with cold symptoms, asking for an antibiotic. The doctor finds the child has a viral infection that won't respond to antibiotics and will get well on its own in a few days regardless of the treatment rendered.

"But *do* something!" the mother pleads.

So the physician may prescribe cough medicine or deconges-
tants that help to relieve the child's symptoms but do nothing
for the viral infection itself. This is a form of placebo treatment,
one that is given in good faith on both sides. Cold symptoms
are relieved and the mother's and child's anxiety is alleviated
because they know the infection isn't serious.

What Makes a Placebo Work?

Is the placebo strictly a psychological phenomenon, then, or
is there some physiologic effect taking place?

This is a hard question to answer. Sometimes the physical
and psychological are intimately intertwined.

A woman came to her doctor complaining of excruciating
ulcer pain. The only thing was, she had no ulcer. Her doctor
decided to try an experiment. He presented her with a large pill
the size of a half dollar. Ceremoniously he dropped the pill into
a glass of water.

"When the fizzing stops," he told her, "sip this slowly. Be
sure you drink every bit of it."

Now, the pill was nothing but effervescent Vitamin C. It had
no curative powers whatsoever. Yet the results were dramatic.
The patient's persistent, debilitating pain was gone almost immediately.

According to this woman's doctor, the single most important
aspect of his treatment was that he held the tablet with a pair of
tweezers. "It gave the impression that the pill was too powerful
for me to touch with my bare hands," he said.

Another example of the placebo effect is the physician's
dress. Recently a number of articles have been written on what
is known as the "white coat syndrome." A patient having his
blood pressure taken by someone in a white coat in a doctor's
office or clinic or hospital setting often becomes anxious. In a
setting such as a grocery store, however, he may well have a
much lower reading.

Think of the advertisements we see on television for various
medical preparations. They often begin with a thoughtful, sin-

cere, distinguished-looking physician in a white coat. Of course he's just an actor, but seeing him in that white coat causes us to sit up and listen when he presents "medical evidence" for his product. His white coat symbolizes the authority, training, and knowledge of the medical profession.

Many practitioners within the alternative health movement have come to realize that the way they present their cures and their titles (real or bogus) has as much or more to do with the patient's recovery as the actual content of the cures.

Put yourself in this patient's place. Your best friend has glowingly recommended that you see an acupuncturist who helped get rid of her headaches which are "just like yours." The last time you went to see your M.D. he seemed distracted and didn't really seem to listen to all your problems like you thought he should. The acupuncturist's office is clean and modern, but you are amazed at the interesting assortment of herbs and other medicines you've never heard of filling the jars along the wall. After your treatments you can still faintly smell the balmy scent of burned mutterer, a leafy herb, he used as part of your treatment. And you think you just might feel a little better—after all, the "doctor" said you would be. This happens everyday to people just like you.

But Is It Right?

The long established medical use of placebos has come under increasing attack from those concerned that it may not be ethical to use them without the patient's knowledge. Placebos necessarily involve some degree of deception, even though it may be benevolent deception. Assuming the attitude that "the doctor knows best," many physicians prescribing placebos have no intention of telling their patients what the situation really is. They figure this is the best way to help their patients. The woman with the conversion reaction who couldn't walk was able to go home and resume her life after taking the sugar pills. She also had an opportunity to continue in outpatient psychotherapy, as she had been doing, rather than being hospitalized.

Yes, the doctor "tricked" her; but it was obviously in her best interests.

Critics beg to differ. They insist that informed consent takes precedence over the physician's determination to act, even when he is convinced that deception is in the best interest of her patient. The patients, critics argue, have the right to know.

The matter of informed consent becomes even more important when we understand that placebos have an effect on more than just a person's mind. They can have a very real effect on the body as well. We're not just talking about suggestible people, either. There is no basic personality difference between those who respond to placebos and those who are unaffected by them. Placebos, you see, can cause the production and release of certain chemicals within a person's body. These chemicals, called endorphins, produce a response similar to that of drugs used to treat pain. The result is a lessening of the patient's pain, all because of the placebo effect.

Principles for Using Placebos

Placebos themselves are neither good nor bad. It all depends upon how they are used. (In alternative medicine, almost any vitamin, pill, potion, or treatment can serve as a placebo.) When it comes to placebos, certain principles should act as guidelines.

1. *The placebo effect should only be used for the benefit of the patient.* A placebo never should be used to legitimize a specific technique. Yet this is exactly what is done within the arena of alternative medicine. For instance, guided imagery and consulting with spirit guides are legitimate, practitioners claim, because they "activate the placebo effect." Certainly, there are many ways to achieve the placebo effect, if that is your goal, without the occultic intrusion of demonic spirit guides.

2. *Placebos should only be used in cases where they really are necessary.* Before a placebo is used, there should be plenty of evidence indicating that it really is necessary.

In many cases within the alternative health movement, the

placebo effect is the most important method of treatment. Even when there are more effective medical treatments available, the placebo is chosen simply because it is natural—and natural, many alternative practitioners believe, just *has* to be better. Since it often isn't a real medicine at all, the placebo effect may be the *only* positive effect.

Now, it might be argued legitimately that a placebo should be prescribed for something such as anxiety. But what about the cough a pneumonia patient has? For a bacterial infection, a patient needs antibiotics—real medicine. It's the only way to eliminate the root cause.

3. *If a patient is to be deceived, the physician should be able to make a sound case for why it is necessary*. Placebo deception may indeed be the best course of action for a particular patient, but a doctor should have a strong reason for doing so, a reason based in reality. The doctor should not be subjecting his patient to his particular religious or philosophical views.

Why is a therapeutic touch practitioner telling her patient she is manipulating unidentified energy fields, when in fact there is no proof energy fields such as this exist at all? What case can a practitioner make for perpetrating such a deception?

Any legitimate observer has the right to ask for evidence that the deception is necessary. And he has a right to expect an honest answer.

4. *A physician should determine whether there is any other condition, either physical or psychological, that might be confused or hidden by the use of a placebo*. It isn't appropriate to use a placebo if it's going to mask another problem that needs to be dealt with. For example, acupunture may be effective in treating certain kinds of headache disorders, but it won't do a thing for a case of appendicitis. Yet if a person has used acupunture to relieve her headaches, she may try to relieve abdominal discomfort the same way. In fact, giving her relief from her pain could kill her if a surgeon does not remove her inflamed, gangrenous appendix.

5. *If using the placebo will require a physician to deceive*

his patient, the physician should carefully consider how the deception will effect the patient. The element of trust between a physician and her patient should never be violated. Otherwise the relationship between the two will be much less effective. Without trust, a physician loses credibility.

Some patients want their physician to do whatever the doctor deems best. But other patients want to be fully informed. They don't take kindly to being deceived or left out of the decision making.

This guideline is not only for physicians. It should also hold for alternative health practitioners. To fail to inform their patients of the full nature of their procedures—including the religious aspects and spiritual implications of some of their practices—violates this basic trust.

Help or Harm?

Some would have us believe that placebos, if not always helpful, at least cause no harm. This is not so. Dr. D. W. Beaven, Professor of Medicine at Christchurch (New Zealand) School of Medicine, states that the Consumers Association, organized by nonmedical lay people in Great Britain, found that although most herbal remedies act as placebos and do very little harm, some substances are toxic.[1] They can be especially dangerous when taken with orthodox medicines to treat serious illnesses. For example, the herbal remedy foxglove has varying amounts of digitalis, a potent heart medicine, in it. If this were to be mixed with other cardiac medications it might cause a heart attack.

The Consumers Association found that the widespread, unsupervised sale of herbal medicines left consumers largely unprotected, particularly from unlicensed remedies whose standards are not reliable.

Dr. Robert Becker, author of *The Body Electric,* and a physician himself, talks of placebos and crystals. Crystals, he says, can have a placebo effect on true believers. "Placebos are great stuff. Crystal healing is fine if you don't have very much wrong with you." But he goes on to caution that seriously ill crystal fanciers who choose crystal therapy over useful medical treatment could find themselves in real trouble. Placebos can only do so much.

Because they sometimes discount the effects of placebos, many medical professionals look upon alternative medical healers as unimportant. Yet, it would be foolish to completely close our minds to placebos. Used appropriately, placebos can be powerful and beneficial.

The Tomato Effect

In the early 1800s, tomatoes were not eaten in North America. Why? Because they were believed to be poisonous. It was obvious. After all, tomatoes belong to the deadly nightshade family. The fact that the French and Italians were eating more and more tomatoes without apparent harm didn't encourage early Americans to try them. It simply did not make sense to eat "poisonous" food.

Then, in 1820, Robert Johnson ate a tomato on the steps of the courthouse in Salem, New Jersey. To everyone's amazement, he survived. The tomato didn't even make him sick. Only then did Americans begin to eat tomatoes—many of them grudgingly. When we speak of "the tomato effect" in medicine, we're talking about a truly effective treatment for a certain disease that is ignored or rejected merely because it does not make sense in light of currently accepted medical practice.[2]

Before we reject an unorthodox treatment we should ask: "Could this be a tomato?" That is, could it be that this treatment is on the forefront of something beneficial?

A wise patient will ask certain questions.

1. *Is this treatment a placebo?* Before accepting a treatment, you should ask whether the treatment is a placebo. A yes answer need not rule the procedure out, but it is something you have a right to know.

2. *Does this treatment require any religious involvement either from me or from the practitioner?* We can accept the surgical removal of an appendix as having no religious intent.

The prescription of an antihypertensive medication to someone with an increased risk of suffering a stroke because of high blood pressure has no religious implications. On the other hand, meditation, guided imagery, spirit channeling, and the manipulation of energy forces are associated with Eastern religions. If you want to be a Hindu or to practice some other type of Eastern religion, do so with your eyes open and by your own choosing. But don't be tricked into participating for so-called medical reasons. There are too many other options for your mortal life and too much else at stake for your immortal soul.

Dealing in Desperation

W. H. Auden wrote in *For the Time Being: A Christmas Oratorio:* "We who must die demand a miracle."

Trading on a currency of fear and undocumented miraculous cures, alternative health practitioners gravitate toward the unfortunate victims of incurable diseases. This happens again and again.

For many people, cancer is the most dreaded of all diseases. Little wonder, then, that New Age health periodicals abound with purported treatments and cures aimed at cancer patients. Evidently their advertising pays off. Up to 50 percent of patients with cancer, we are told, will consult an alternative healer during the course of their treatment.

The Laetrile controversy of the late '70s and early '80s was a classic example of the desperation of cancer victims on which greed can feed. Loudly proclaiming patients' rights and freedom of choice, Laetrile supporters were successful in convincing large numbers of American cancer patients—78,000 of them by 1978, we are told—that this was indeed a miracle cure. Never mind the opposition of almost every reputable cancer specialist in the country, the Federal Drug Administration, and all major medical organizations. Thousands of Americans left the country to receive Laetrile treatments in Mexico. Parents by the hundreds fled over the border with their sick children, each mom and dad longing for a miracle.

Vast sums of money were involved. In 1979, Laetrile was a

billion dollar a year business. Even after the National Institute of Health and the FDA again provided irrefutable and conclusive evidence in 1982 that the drug was worthless, Laetrile continued to be a windfall industry.

One fraudulent health promoter in Connecticut advertised a medical pill which he claimed would cure cancer. Evidently there were many people desperate enough and sufficiently discouraged with scientific medicine to respond. The man reportedly received more than 1.5 million dollars. When postal inspectors called him to investigate, his top secret ingredient was forcibly unmasked. It was nothing more than sugar. The operator of the scheme was charged, tried, and sentenced to a lengthy prison term in a federal penitentiary.

The real salvation of the alternative health movement, however, may well be the increasing numbers of persons infected with the Acquired Immune Deficiency Syndrome (AIDS). According to Marian Segal of the Federal Drug Administration, AIDS is a "quack's dream come true."[3] Congressional hearings estimate that over 1 billion dollars is spent annually on fraudulent AIDS treatments. The incurable and invariably fatal nature of this disease leads to incredible fear and desperation on the part of patients and of their families and friends as well. They will try almost anything and pay almost any price for even a glimmer of hope.

Citing excessive red tape in the development of promising new drugs, and hinting at political and moral prejudice against AIDS patients, "guerrilla clinics" have sprung up to meet the demand for treatment at any price. Blue-green algae, thymus gland thumping, herbal therapy, macrobiotics, bathing in chlorine bleach, bee pollen, injections of hydrogen peroxide, thymus gland extract, even injections of a patient's own urine—these are among the worthless and often harmful treatments being offered AIDS patients in the name of free choice and holistic health.

The amazing thing is that for every treatment, a satisfied customer is ready to step forward and testify to its success. Such is the strength of denial in these patients who want so deeply to be healed. Such is the power of the placebo.

FAITH HEALING

I seriously doubt that any of us would argue with the conclusion that it's wrong to sell sugar pills promoted as miracle cures through the mail. Why, then, do so many insist that it's all right to promote unscientific, unproven medical practices in a church?

The placebo effect can be a powerful influence in faith healing. In a study related by Elizabeth Gettig from Western Pennsylvania Hospital in Pittsburgh, a faith healer was to pray for three hospitalized patients.[4] The patients knew nothing about the prayer, and they didn't improve at all. The healer was then dismissed from the case and his healing efforts stopped. At this point the physician involved informed the patients that a faith healer was praying for them though he had long since stopped. Immediately all three patients experienced a lessening of their symptoms. The conclusion was that it was the psychological effect of the patient's expectations that was responsible for their sense of improvement.

An evangelist named Peter Popoff came to San Francisco on a faith healing crusade. He warned his audience about the "terrible doctors who are asking you to put chemicals into your bodies." He yelled out: "Doctor Jesus doesn't use any chemicals!" Then he had the ill and infirm come forward and throw their medications on the stage. These discarded medications included such lifesaving substances as nitroglycerine tablets, insulin, and vitally needed heart medicines.[5]

An excited ten-year-old boy came to the crusade on crutches, convinced he would walk out on two strong, healthy legs. His faith in Christ's ability to heal him through Popoff was unquestioning. But when the crusade ended, the little fellow left—still crippled and still on crutches. His enthusiasm gone, tears streamed down his cheeks. Who had let this boy down—God or Popoff?

Popoff was a fraud. He used a hidden radio device through which his wife whispered to him from backstage. She got her information from "prayer cards" people filled out beforehand, and from her own conversations with them before the meeting began. Popoff, however, proclaimed it all as divine messages from God.

Popoff repeatedly "healed" one man, who had been planted by investigators, at different meetings—of diseases he didn't have. Once, disguised as a woman, he was even "healed" of uterine cancer.

Christians who believe in the literal interpretation of the Bible believe in miracles. The authors of this book certainly do. Consider the miracles of Jesus Christ. He healed lepers (Matt. 8). He gave sight to the blind (Matt. 9). He restored a withered hand (Matt. 12). He miraculously fed 5,000 people (Luke 9). He walked on water (Matt. 14). He healed a deaf mute (Mark 7). He even raised the dead (John 11, Luke 7, Mark 5).

So, then, if we believe in miracles, what are we to make of the miraculous healings proposed by those within the alternative health movement (including so-called Christian faith healers)?

St. Augustine said, "Miracles do not happen in contradiction to nature, but only in contradiction to that which is known to us of nature." He may be right in most cases. Routine coronary artery bypass surgery, in which blood vessels are grafted around blockages and blood flow is restored to diseased areas of the heart, gives new life to thousands of people every year. In many ways this is a miracle.

Medicines such as penicillin were termed "miracle drugs" when they first came out because they were so effective at fighting deadly diseases that had previously taken millions of lives. Today's medical miracles are tomorrow's mainstream treatments.

But Christ's raising of people from the dead was something

quite different. It was miraculous in His day, and now 2,000 years later it is still miraculous. Many modern-day faith healers would have us believe that their "miracles" fall into the same supernatural category as that of Christ's.

Hank Hanegraff, of the Christian Research Institute, writes: "If the New Age movement is the greatest threat to evangelical Christianity from without, I believe the word-faith or 'positive confession' movement may well be considered its greatest threat from within."[6] This rapidly growing and influential movement offers the idea that everyone can be financially prosperous and physically healthy. The key to this supposedly unlimited health and wealth? Faith, exercised as a tool to compel God to provide whatever you want.

"You can have what you say."

"Faith is not something which we have so much as it is something that we do."

"The reason you haven't been healed is that you don't have enough faith."

Promises of perfect health? Personal responsibility for your own illness and that of your families? Sounds a lot like New Age medicine with its farfetched and usually unprovable claims of miraculous healing—ideas like "create your own reality," and personal guilt for any sickness. (Red flags flying high!) It would appear that many have been misled by the tantalizing lure of perfect health.

Yes, God honors faith (Matt. 9:29; James 1:6–8). But no, God does not promise perfect health. He points to the prophets of the Old Testament as "an example of suffering and patience" (James 5:10), and the prophets, we're told, were destitute, afflicted, beaten, tortured, and executed (Heb. 12:36–37). Certainly they were not examples of perfect health; yet they are acclaimed as having tremendous faith.

I agree with Elliot Miller, author of *Healing: Does God Always Heal?* that one of the most disturbing aspects of the "faith movement" is its similarity to the "mind science" movement typified by Christian Science and Unity School of Christianity. Both of these groups strongly believe (1) in the denial of illness, (2) that it is always God's will that we are physically perfect, and (3) that by simply affirming your desires you can create your own experience either positively or negatively.

Statements and attitudes like, "I've been healed, it's just that the symptoms are still hanging on," have led to much unnecessary suffering and even in some cases needless death. Followers of the "faith movement" or the "positive confession" movement may well be Christians, but they are misled and in error both physically and spiritually when they *demand* healing from God.

For them, faith has become a tool, a force with which to create the desires of their minds. And God, whom they claim to serve, has become their servant. God does not have to do anything. Hank Hanegraff says it well: "The Creator is the Lord of the universe, not a cosmic 'gofer' at the beck and call of His creation."

The Christian Responsibility

If the Christian community is to retain its credibility, it must rise up in anger and disgust, ridding itself of those who promote health fraud in the name of God and Jesus Christ.

I submit that Christians can define miracles as the striking or unusual workings by which God intervenes supernaturally in our world for the purpose of achieving His larger purpose. When viewed in this light, the miracles of the Bible—primarily associated with the spreading of the gospel of Jesus Christ and the teaching and preaching of God's Word—clearly become distinguished from the world of magic and sorcery.

Biblical miracles are clustered around three distinct periods in history:

1. *The exodus of the children of Israel from Egypt and their wilderness wanderings*. Moses was given the miraculous ability to do signs and wonders, which convinced the people that God was with them and working through them—the parting of the Red Sea, providing manna from heaven, and water in the desert are examples.

2. *The prophetic days of Elijah and Elisha.* These prophets lived at a time when the very worship of the Israelites was at stake. These miracles included a dramatic encounter between the prophets of Baal and Elijah, who had prophesied a three-and-a-half year drought. The confrontation culminated when Elijah called fire from heaven which completely consumed his thoroughly water soaked altar, including the stones themselves and the ground it sat upon. The drought was ended by the miraculous intervention of God (1 Kings 18).

3. *The time of Christ and the apostles.* Christ performed many miracles, some of which we have already mentioned. The greatest miracle of all was His own personal resurrection from the dead. After His ascension to heaven, the apostles performed miracles as they introduced Christianity to the world.

Each of these periods was important to the accomplishment of God's purposes for the Hebrew people, the Christian church, and the entire world. They had three main aims: to glorify God, to establish the supernatural basis of God's message, and to meet human needs. They provide us with the assurance that God is present and active in the lives of Christians, that whatever happens to us is of concern to God, and that nothing occurs by chance.

While today there may be the occasional demonstration of God's power in unusual ways for special purposes, the chief emphasis in the Bible is on God's constant power in working through humans who follow the way of ordered nature.

God is sovereign and can cure. Often He does it by working through recognized treatments. If we do not take advantage of the medical opportunities presented us, perhaps we are testing God.

When Jesus was being tempted by Satan, He *did not* choose to test God by jumping off the cliff (Matt. 4:1–11). Yes, God certainly had the power to save Jesus if He had jumped, but to have *demanded* that God save Him would have put Jesus in the decision-making seat. That is what the original temptation of man was, and that is what it continues to be: "You can be in charge. You can make this happen. You can be like God." It is the line of reasoning used both by the New Age and by some Christian healers who want to totally control their destiny.

Because of our country's stand on the separation of church and state, it is difficult for the federal government to intervene in church-promoted methods, however bogus they may be. "Religious freedom!" both Christian and New Age promoters shout.

It behooves every church to police its own members. We have a responsibility to examine what kinds of practices our churches are promoting in the name of God and Christ. And as consumers, we have a responsibility to tread carefully, knowledgeably, and wisely. It seems that as quickly as new, highly questionable treatments are investigated and their true worthlessness exposed, along comes another variation of the same thing. Different name, fresh promoter, new gimmick, but the same old worthless stuff nevertheless. Some of these promoters use words meant to strike a responsive note in Christians—such as "Son-shine." Some of the promoters work through churches and Christian organizations. Some of the gimmicks are designed to have special appeal to the Christian community—fish symbols, for example, or doves.

Chapter Ten

WHERE DO WE GO FROM HERE?

$\mathbf{M}$arie and Toni, two Christian women, live in a town of about 25,000 people where everyone knows everyone else's business.

When Rose, an attractive, outgoing woman, moved into town and began attending the main Protestant church, she was given a warm welcome. By all appearances, here was a woman who seemed to be everything a good Christian should be. She also happened to be a marketer for a multilevel company that sold herbs and vitamins, with miraculous claims about all products.

Before long, the pastor was one of Rose's clients. In fact, virtually all the church leaders were soon buying her products. Rose went to women's Bible study and made friends with the ladies there. She followed up on her new friends and, one by one, managed to get them involved in the practice of herbal medicine. Using iridology and muscle testing (applied kinesiology), she would diagnose their health problems and suggest a course of treatment. Soon Rose was much too busy running her business to attend the Bible study.

Not only were people buying from Rose, but quite a few

219

church members became deeply involved in selling her products at church gatherings. At a church-sponsored young mothers group, for instance, Rose—who billed herself as a "nutritional counselor"—gave her testimony about how God had used her practice of diet and supplements to "change her life." And, she added, through iridology and applied kinesiology, she could help each person find out just which herbs he or she needed.

Rose also taught about "energy blocks" in the body. Not to worry, though. She could check for any blockages and alter them simply by passing her hands over a person's body. Rose sold a device she called a "diode," which was supposed to rebalance or filter out negative energy.

Marie and Toni were not impressed. They did some research and discovered that everything this woman was doing was totally unscientific and ineffectual. Rose's only credentials came from the fact that she had taken a training course through the multilevel marketing firm that employed her—the one that sold the vitamins and herbal products.

So Marie and Toni gathered together information on the various practices Rose was teaching, and presented it to the church board. Their response? "Stay out of this and keep quiet, or the church will have to discipline you." You see, several board members and their wives were deeply involved with Rose and her program.

After several months of frustration, Marie and her family left their church. Several months later, Toni and her family also left. "We had to," Marie explained sadly. "We could not accept the 'nutritianity' that had taken over the church."

Certainly there was a problem with Rose's selling techniques. But even worse were her attempts to diagnose. When the pastor's sister despaired about her newborn son who was being treated in the intensive care unit for a serious neonatal condition, Rose pressured the woman to bring the baby home so Rose could treat the infant with herbs.

In fact, a good many of her sales were made through appeals to mothers to, "Do what's right for your children."

"Herbs," Rose said, "are God's food."

One mother took her son to Rose for an evaluation. Based on his "iris patterns," Rose predicted the boy would have a predilection to sexual perversion. Can you imagine the impact of telling this little fellow that he was going to be a sexual pervert? It's hard to imagine anything more insensitive or cruel.

"The church is a unique market for sales techniques like Rose's," Toni noted. It is for many alternative health techniques. It's a safe market.

"Everyone figures Christians don't lie," Toni explained. "You can depend on a fellow Christian to tell you the truth. When Rose told people herbs would cure them, they believed her."

"The family concept of the church protected her," Marie added. "You aren't supposed to air your dirty laundry outside the church family."

In the end, church leaders were forced to admit the problems with Rose's methods. She was told she had to quit selling her products on church property. Neither could she talk about her products at church gatherings. Still, the leaders refused to make any statement about the false and fraudulent practices of iridology and energy manipulation. Ultimately, rather than change her practices, Rose chose to move on to another church where she continues to conduct her herbal products business to this day.

Rose billed her business as a "Christian nutritional counseling service," which would imply that it is based on biblical principles. Yet, as we all know, biblical principles do not support iridology or energy manipulation or health fraud.

Thanks to Marie and Toni's persistence, guidelines for assessing iridology and other alternative health care techniques were brought out by the church's denominational governing board. It was only a partial victory, however. Rather than condemn iridology as an unscientific practice, the written statement, signed by an associate director of the board, read, "The client has the responsibility to determine if the iridologist's concept of holistic has a Christian frame of reference or a New Age frame of reference."[1] In other words, if a Christian performs iridology, it's okay. Otherwise, it's not okay. (Red flag No. 12 flies high once again.) This prestigious group, responsible for church doctrine, chose to skate around the issue. What will you decide to do?

WE MUST BE DISCERNING

Unfortunately, well-meaning Christians often fall prey to those who use Scripture to back up their claims. Iridologists, for instance, quote such passages as Matthew 6:22–23 and Luke 11:34, 36 ("The lamp of the body is the eye . . ."). Marie and Toni's church board did say this interpretation was open to serious question and could mislead immature Christians into thinking that iridology is sanctioned in Scripture.

Let's get something straight. Not only is iridology not a *Christian* method, it is not an accurate diagnostic method at all. *It is nothing but health fraud*. A fraudulent practice is a fraudulent practice, whether it is associated with the New Age movement or with the Christian church.

Not only was Rose committing medical fraud, she was promoting spiritual fraud as well. Rose pushed her nutritional theories as being "God's way" to health, and supported the claims for iridology with the work of an elderly California chiropractor, Bernard Jensen.

Dr. Jensen has been one of the leaders of the alternative health movement for years. His self-published book *A New Lifestyle For Health and Happiness* promotes the same unproven and unscientific methods that Rose was using. Perhaps Rose failed to recognize Jensen's affinity for occult and Eastern religious practices.

Among others, Jensen dedicated his book to Ernest Holmes, founder of the think-yourself-well United Church of Religious Science; to Harry Edwards, a medium who communicated with dead scientists such as Pasteur and Lister as spirit guides; and Sai Baba, an Indian guru who claims to be the reincarnation of several Hindu deities as well as Jesus Christ.

In the alternative medicine, health fraud and spiritual fraud walk hand in hand. How many of Rose's Christian clients recognized the occult and Eastern religious undertones of her advice? Alternative medicine, with its "natural" methods and holistic smile, deceives many, both medically and spiritually.

Yet we all have spiritual needs. Should medical doctors recognize people's spiritual aspects so they can better treat their physical bodies?

A CHALLENGE TO MEDICAL DOCTORS

To their credit, those in the alternative health care movement have long recognized and openly acknowledged the spiritual aspects of persons—although much of what they claim as spiritual is a deceptive counterfeit of biblical concepts of Christianity. On the other hand, established medicine has basically ignored the spiritual aspects of patients in its training of physicians, nurses, and other care-givers. This attitude throws the door wide open to alternative practitioners. Luke 11:24–26 reminds us that a spiritual vacuum will be filled, and if it is not filled with God, then that vacuum is open to evil.

Christian physicians have to share some of the blame as well. We, too, have largely abandoned our patients spiritually. One reason is that the majority of physicians are unaware of the false message of the alternative health movement. We're unfamiliar with the practices, the techniques, and the philosophies that underpin its workings. Instead, we need to recognize them as the health and soul robbers they are.

I conducted a poll of physicians in the Christian Medical Society here in Austin. In general, the physicians—who represent a wide variety of specialities—weren't aware that their patients were involved in alternative health practices. This is interesting, since I find that many of my patients are either involved or clearly interested in these questionable methods, and my experience is not unusual. A study done at the pediatric oncolgy clinics of M. D. Anderson Cancer Center found that 39 percent of the patients and parents interviewed had either tried, considered, or received recommendations for unproven remedies.

Another study gives us these statistics: 67 percent of Americans now believe in the supernatural, 42 percent believe they have been in contact with the dead, and 23 percent believe in reincarnation—philosophies of alternative health care practitioners like Bernie Siegel, which are forbidden by the Bible.[2]

When medical doctors are confronted by patients treading close to or actually involved in non-traditional practices, we are often uncomfortable with the subject. We often shy away without asking questions. Or we assume a superior or paternal air. Our actions, if not our voices, shout out: "How can you believe something so ridiculous?" Degrading our patients does not help us understand the needs and desires that are leading them to alternative health practices.

But, you may ask, if medical doctors must recognize their patients' spiritual needs, then why not incorporate alternative health practices into the main stream of medicine?

ALTERNATIVE *AND* SCIENTIFIC MEDICINE?

Many individuals and groups seek the merger of alternative medicine and scientific medicine as we know it today. Naturopaths, "holistic" M.D.s, shamans, political action groups, New Age churches, many chiropractors, and thousands of patients are all supporters of alternative medicine. Many others, including the influential World Health Organization, voice their support for a merger of alternative and established medicine.

In an address before a holistic health conference sponsored by the Association for Holistic Health, David Harris, speaker, director and association president, said, "We have been accused of contaminating science with religion. I just want to say that we see the marriage of science with religion as bringing about the next stage of our evolution."

Olga Worrall, a psychic healer and speaker at this same medical conference, said, "I believe that science and religion are going to have a love affair and are going to get married."

Other New Age practitioners, like Michael Harner, a modern-day shaman, are proposing this blending:

There is no conflict between shamanic practice and modern medicine. . . . One day, and I hope soon, a modern version of the shaman will work side-by-side with orthodox western physicians. . . . Equally exciting is the prospect of physicians being trained in shamanic methods of healing so they can combine both approaches in their practice.[3]

An exciting prospect? We don't think so. Shamanic practices, as we have seen in this book, are nothing more than occultic practices that lead to spiritual deception.

It is dangerous to blend proven, scientific medicine with many alternative health practices. For by accepting them, we are by implication accepting a non-science into an area of science. By dabbling in the alternatives, we are giving credence to unproven, unscientific health practices that delude, confuse, cheat, and even kill countless people each year.

Thankfully not everyone is pleased about this proposed wedding. Because the nature of the doctor/patient relationship involves a kind of trust or submission to the healer, there is an opportunity for the healer—whether physician, nurse, or alternative practitioner—to project his feelings onto his patient. Thoughtful people are asking whether they want to submit themselves to this kind of influence from unscientific sources.

GOOD OLD DAYS OF MEDICINE

As we have seen, certain basic New Age principles spring up again and again. One of these principles is a spiritual world view that pervades the entire alternative health industry, and it definitely is not in line with Christianity.

Brooks Alexander, of the Spiritual Counterfeits Project, agrees. He writes:

The overriding commitment of these new scientists is not to science in the traditional sense of the term, but to the propagation of an essentially religious world view by manipulating the prestige, apparatus, and artifacts of scientific knowledge.

Many alternative healers yearn for a return to the "good old days" of medicine. It's not Norman Rockwell's idea of old-time doctors they want, mind you. They long for the bone rattling, chanting witch doctor dancing around a sick patient to the beat of an animal skin drum. Just listen to Colonel Johnny M. Lamb, Chairman of the Department of Surgery, and Residency Program Director at Travis Air Force Base: "I propose that by getting in touch with the Shamanistic, intuitive side of ourselves, we have the best chance to bring our society that heritage from the past that will allow us more potency."[5]

An article in the *Journal of Health and Social Behavior* (Volume 28, 1987), quotes a study which compares mainstream family physicians with alternative physicians—ones who use techniques most doctors would regard as lacking in scientific justification or efficacy. Not only did the alternative doctors express a good deal of dissatisfaction and disillusionment with mainstream medicine; a majority of them reported they had undergone intense personal experiences which had shaped their feeling about medicine and their practice of it. In fact, undefined religious and/or spiritual experiences were reported by twenty-two of the thirty respondents.

Said one holistic doctor, "I realized I had to live my life as I wanted to . . . [I had] a spiritual awakening . . . I became aware of the intuitive qualities in myself. I joined the Church of Religious Science, was very active for a few years. They have something called 'spiritual mind treatment.' It's making a religious affirmation, a commitment. I use it and I use it in my practice."

Almost one-half of the holistic physicians reported that personal experiences with their own illness, or that of close family members, had been influential in leading to their current holistic stance. One said, "Which influence was most important to me? Having nearly died. It made me face the life I had lived. On my death bed, that opened the door. I saw I was hungry for life."

In summation, the article stated: "These holistic physicians appeared to have been influenced greatly by subjective, highly personal experiences which took place outside the world of medicine."

If the New Age world view of alternative medicine becomes intermingled with the medical community and takes root there, it gets harder and harder to weed out. It becomes more accepted. People stop questioning it. The insurance companies pay for it. Medicare quits arguing, and picks up the tab. In the end, you and I are the ones who may ultimately be asked to support this non-Christian world view.

IS THERE A MIDDLE GROUND?

Can we address the issues of body, mind, and spirit without going overboard in one direction or another? Can we be scientific without worshiping the mind? Can we be spiritual without becoming like those who abandon the physical, emotional, or mental aspects of man in favor of the spiritual alone?

The answer is Yes, there is a middle ground.

Despite its insistence that it is a truly holistic health movement, alternative medicine does not really provide a balanced approach to either physical medicine or spiritual medicine. It often presents us with an overemphasis of metaphysical spirituality without recognizing the physical and emotional impact of diseases as well. Its rejection of modern scientific methods negates the potential good of recognizing the emotional aspects of illness. In very few cases can the approach of the alternative medicine movement be termed balanced.

The Role of the Modern Physician

Whenever I describe my work as a family physician, people always say, "There aren't many like you around anymore!" Nothing could be further from the truth. There are many family physicians today. The problem is that through the years there has been an overemphasis on specialization within the medical

educational community. Specialists have been held in high esteem both by the public and in medical schools.

Today's well-trained physician, whether a more highly spe-
cialized neurosurgeon or a more broadly trained family physician, has the responsibility to provide his or her patient with
the best medical care currently available. The general public
senses the need for more than just technical excellence, however. There is also a demand that the patient be recognized as a
person—a whole person, with feelings, individual needs, and
personal preferences. The complete physician must recognize
and work with patients to educate, to communicate, to understand them as a person.

Today we have a real tension between what medicine provides and what patients demand: They want the finest technology delivered by the best physicians—but they also want their
doctors to behave as though it were still the 1920s, when what
we did best was offer understanding, compassion, and support.

It's not that we *can't* have both. It's that physicians and patients alike have come to expect that we *won't* have both—that
somehow compassion, understanding, and support for the patient goes out when high-tech medicine comes in. This is unfortunate indeed. It drives our patients right into the waiting arms
of those who appear less antiseptic and more human.

What, then, should the family physician do to deal with the
spiritual aspects of illness?

First of all, a physician should never "bend" the truth or promote unproven methods just to prove a spiritual point. Any
method based in deception should be rejected, such as iridology or applied kinesiology and others which have been scientifically proven to be ineffective. Suggesting questionable nutrition practices because it's "God's way" or "God's food" is in
most cases both scientifically and spiritually deceptive. Promoting unproven methods must be clearly presented as experimental.

Second, the source of any health practitioner's ideas and
methods involving spirituality should be clearly revealed to the

patient. Christian physicians and others should make clear the biblical origin of their advice to patients in spiritual matters. Support of alternative medical practices such as visualization and spirit guides derived from the *Tibetan Book of the Dead* should be just as obvious. Those reading *Dr. Dean Ornish's Program for Reversing Heart Disease* have a right to be aware of his belief in the yoga philosophy as taught by Swami Satchidananda[6] and its influence on his conclusions and suggested methods. Patients have a right to clearly understand a practitioner's spiritual orientation when receiving such treatment.

Proper Licensing for Alternative Practitioners

Mandatory licensing of anyone who provides health care to the public is in the interest of all of us. This would allow for a clear definition of a health provider's scope of practice. Proper licensing is also welcomed by many within the alternative health movement who recognize its validity.

Unfortunately, certain groups like the Coalition for Alternatives in Nutrition and Health Care, called "medical freedom fighters" by *East-West* magazine, stand firmly against the licensing of nutritionists and other health practitioners. Led by Dr. Catherine Frompovich, who has an unaccredited Ph.D. in nutrition and holistic health science from Columbia Pacific University in San Rafael, California, this group opposes legislation to prohibit medical quackery, to fluoridate water, and to prevent the use of fraudulent medical devices. They are also against mandatory vaccinations for communicable diseases. Evidently Dr. Frompovich and others like her don't worry about the American public being at the mercy of poorly trained practitioners of unproven treatments. Their goal is to throw the door wide open to the forced payment of millions of dollars to these "healers" using federal and private insurance funds.

Could Dr. Frompovich have ulterior motives? Let's look at her credentials. The so-called university that awarded her a Ph.D. is a nonaccredited establishment that promotes unproven health practices. Dr. Frompovich, a former "nutritional consultant," would not be allowed to practice if she were required to be a licensed dietitian.

Let's contrast that with the accreditation of someone like Sharon, the coauthor of this book, who holds a Ph.D., an R.D. (registered dietitian), and an L.D. (a licensed dietitian). To achieve her Ph.D. degree, Sharon was required to take postgraduate classes and do research for four full years (with no summer break). She passed both written and oral tests and finally received a Master of Science degree after two full years of on-site study, and a Ph.D. in nutrition after four full years of on-site study.

To become a registered dietitian, a title designated by the American Dietetic Association, Sharon took a rigorous written examination to test her knowledge and understanding of nutrition and dietetics. The designation licensed dietitian (L.D.) is established within each state to designate persons whom the state deems qualified to give nutritional care.

David Stewart and Henry Spille, educators and authors of the book *Diploma Mills: Degrees of Fraud,* point out the real danger lies in "diploma mills" that grant degrees with requirements that "emulate" but are actually far less demanding than those at legitimate colleges and universities.

No wonder Frompovich and others like her so vigorously attack health care regulation. Yet to whom should you entrust your physical health?

We'd like to see proper licensing for all health care practitioners. Licensing would provide consumer protection from fraudulent practitioners with dubious educational backgrounds. It would also provide a means of regulating health providers who exceed the limitations of their training—by sanctions or the removal of their licenses to practice.

Governmental agencies have a responsibility to act in the interest of the public welfare. Individual citizens have a right to receive competent medical care from carefully regulated and supervised providers. Unfortunately, some groups, upon receiving licensing, would no doubt point to this as governmental approval and proof of efficacy even when no such proof exists. To avoid this travesty, scientific proof of efficacy should be a requirement for all health care providers to be licensed.

We admit that this won't solve all the problems of health fraud and quackery, but it will give health officials some control over those who use, abuse, and maybe even kill their patients.

WHAT DOES THE FUTURE HOLD?

Is alternative medicine and its amalgamation of false spirituality really the wave of the future? Will we indeed see a time when a shaman is on the staff of every hospital in our nation? Are we destined to see meditative exercises broadcast over the television sets in hospital rooms? Will we do away with licensing and accept minimal education for various practitioners? Will we cease to enforce mandatory vaccinations against communicable diseases and needlessly endanger the lives of our children? Are we in fact headed for a time when quackery will again kill a larger number of Americans than all the diseases it pretends to cure? Not if physicians and patients will take more responsibility for proper health care and will educate themselves about these deceptive practices.

The Physician's Responsibilities

As physicians, we have a responsibility to listen to our patients. We need to answer their questions and to anticipate their fears. We need to touch our patients and show them our concern. We also need to consider our possible overreliance on technological advances. Not only are patients paying a terribly high price for this technology; we physicians are alienating many by the magnitude and cost incurred in test after test.

We have a responsibility to provide the best possible care and to stay abreast of medical advances which can benefit our patients. Good medical care will only be enhanced by treating each of our patients as an individual and not just another gallbladder or diabetic that walks through the door. Willingness to communicate, listen, and allow for input from the patient will work wonders in healing the rift between physicians and their patients.

We physicians have a responsibility to address the issue of medical access for all persons in our country. It's time we face reality and recognize that many in America don't have access to adequate medical care. Furthermore, we need to stop looking at our patients as potential adversaries. Despite the fact that lawsuits do come, we need to be willing to respond to hurting people, to be reminded of the reasons we went to medical school in the first place. We need to be filled with feelings of renewed compassion for our fellow man. These are our responsibilities.

The Patient's Responsibilities

Patients, you have responsibilities too. You have a responsibility to listen and to read discerningly. You need to learn to separate fact from fiction. We have included a quick reference on page 235, a summary of the alternative therapies, which answers three vital questions: Is the therapy scientifically proven? Medically safe? Spiritually sound? This will enable you to have a quick overview of alternative health care practices.

You also need to be willing to speak up and voice your concerns and questions, to pursue until you get the answers you need. On the other hand, you need to be careful not to become so demanding that your demands interfere with your doctor's ability to meet your needs. You need to consider the benefits of having a primary care physician who can direct and guide your health care in this ever complex and complicated day of medical advances and technology.

With regards to the medical liability crisis, patients need to understand that there can be no 100 percent guaranteed success in every circumstance. Perfect health is not an American right. It's not a God-given right, either.

Spiritual Discernment

The times in which we live do not lessen our responsibility. Paul warned us about times like these: "Now the Spirit expressly says that in latter times some will depart from the faith, giving heed to deceiving spirits and doctrines of devils" (1 Tim. 4:1).

God also warns us: "And the person who turns after mediums and familiar spirits, to prostitute himself with them, I will set My face against that person and cut him off from his people. Sanctify yourselves therefore, and be holy, for I am the LORD your God. And you shall keep My statutes, and perform them" (Lev. 20:6–8).

Today, as in the days of the Old Testament, there are those among us who have trouble resisting the allure of the occult. It's easy to sit here and say how foolish people are to become involved in practices which are blatantly occultic. Yet Paul himself warned in 2 Corinthians 11:14–15: "Satan himself transforms himself into an angel of light. Therefore, it is no great thing if his ministers also transform themselves into ministers of righteousness."

It is up to us to be spiritually discerning. John reminds us:

Beloved, do not believe every spirit, but test the spirits, whether they are of God; because many false prophets have gone out into the world. By this you know the Spirit of God: Every spirit that confesses that Jesus Christ has come in the flesh is of God, and every spirit that does not confess that Jesus Christ has come in the flesh is not of God (1 John 4:1–3).

It's not simply a matter of believing that Jesus is from God. James tells us, "You believe that there is one God. You do well. Even the demons believe—and tremble!" (James 2:19). No, we need to believe and accept the truth that Jesus is indeed "the way, the truth and the life," that no man comes to God except through Him (see John 14:6). We must understand and believe that Jesus is the only Son of God and that salvation comes through Him alone.

In *Healing at Any Price?* Samuel Pfeifer, M.D., says, that venturing into the field of holistic health is like going into a combat area that is filled with booby traps that are apt to blow up without warning at any time. What a dangerous path to tread!

A GENTLE EXHORTATION

Not everyone who becomes involved in potentially danger-ous alternative medical practices is guilty of heresy. Many Chris-tians have been tricked. Others are simply ignorant of the medical facts. We should not be afraid to gently challenge an-other person's religious beliefs and to endeavor to understand them better, even if these beliefs seem to be based on supersti-tion. Each of us needs to become skilled at listening, skilled at understanding, skilled at discussing our faith.

It is not our right to march out on a witch hunt and pro-nounce everything all good or all bad. Natural foods are a good example. Many people prefer to serve these to their family and guests. And certainly there is a valid scientific reason to avoid certain foods (such as those high in fats) in favor of fresh fruits, vegetables, and grains. On the other hand, going overboard in the area of nutrition and embracing macrobiotics, for instance, veers from this healthy pursuit and takes us into dangerous waters.

We need never be poisoned by medical practices contami-nated with false teachings and dangerous techniques. We have the antidote. All we need is a large portion of knowledge, mixed with a healthy dose of discernment, sprinkled liberally with a good bit of common sense, and covered with prayer.

If we band together, we can prevent the return of the witch doctor with his hidden agenda.

Appendix

ALTERNATIVE HEALTH CARE PRACTICES

Natural Therapies

Ayurveda—an ancient healing system from India which blends medical treatments (primarily herbal) with Hindu religious and philosophical concepts.

> Scientific validity (SV)—folk medicine approach largely supplanted in India by modern Western medicine.
>
> Spiritual concerns (SC)—inseparable from Hindu teachings and used to introduce people to Transcendental Meditation.

Bodywork

Massage Therapy—manipulation of muscles by hand for relief of strain and tension.

> SV—a sound part of established physical therapy.
>
> SC—many therapists and schools promote unproven energy manipulation techniques which ascribe to the New Age all-is-one concept of monism.

Rolfing—a care system based on deep connective tissue manipulation.

> SV—limited scientific evidence, may be painful.
>
> SC—the founder and some practitioners influenced by yoga.

Trager Work—a combination of mental and muscular manipulation via a meditative state of altered consciousness.

235

SV—no scientific studies to support its use.

SC—requires both the patient and the therapist to enter the altered state of consciousness called the "hookup."

Chiropractic Medicine—a system of health care based on manipulation of the spine and muscles to treat disease.

SC—a large percentage of chiropractors are involved in New Age medical practices. Some may view their care as a form of energy manipulation.

Colonics—irrigation of the large intestine to remove toxins as a way of maintaining and improving health.

SV—no evidence to support the concept of toxins and deaths have been reported due to this therapy.

SC—none.

Herbalism—medical treatment based entirely on the use of medicinal plants.

SV—numerous modern medications derived from plants. No evidence that herbal remedies offer improvement over modern medications. Reports of contamination and poor quality control within this largely unregulated industry.

SC—few, though some elements of nature worship and communication with plant "spirits" within the broad scope of herbalism.

Homeopathy—a treatment based on the concept that the more dilute a medicine, the more potent.

SV—no conclusive evidence of results beyond placebo effect. Some treatments so dilute as to be only water.

SC—implies treatment through the "spiritual" qualities of its medicines and manipulation of universal energy.

Macrobiotics—a rigid diet and life-style based on Taoist concepts.

SV—if not carried to dangerous extremes, the low-fat diet could have beneficial effects on your health; however, cases of nutritional deficiency have occurred. No evidence of cancer cures as claimed by its promoters.

SC—an all-consuming life-style based on an Oriental religious philosophy with a meditative altered state of consciousness encouraged while eating. Promotes planetary unity through its dietary program.

Osteopathy—a complete system of medical care based on established scientific treatment with additional emphasis on care of musculo-skeletal problems through manipulative therapy.

> SV—fully licensed for the practice of all types of medical care. Research documentation of the effectiveness of manipulative therapy for a limited number of health problems.

> SC—as with all sorts of health practitioners some have become heavily involved in highly questionable New Age medical methods.

Mind Therapies

Biofeedback—a technique for gaining some measure of control over certain bodily functions through the visual or auditory response of a machine connected to that function.

> SV—well-established uses for specific physical problems such as control of headaches and blood pressure.

> SC—often misunderstood and misused within the alternative medicine movement. Often used to justify and lend credence to various "mind over matter" therapies.

Christian Science—a religion founded by Mary Baker Eddy based on a denial of disease, sin, and death which are viewed by her followers as mental illusions.

> SV—no scientific evidence of the healing claims of the church or its various "practitioners." Numerous deaths, especially of children, documented as a result of failure to seek proper medical care.

> SC—a completely unbiblical religious doctrine including the denial of sin, evil, Christ's resurrection among others.

Dreamwork—a theory that analysis of one's dreams can lead to an understanding of the subconscious.

> SV—strongly promoted by Carl Jung and his followers, dream analysis is one tool among many used by modern mental health workers.

> SC—potential for abuse as the interpretations are based on the biases of the interpreter. Used by some to promote occultic contact with spirit entities completely contrary to biblical warning.

Hypnosis—the inducement of a trancelike state of heightened suggestibility or compliance.

SV—use is well documented in numerous medical settings including anesthesia and psychiatry.

SC—involves an altered state of consciousness in which the person being hypnotized is vulnerable to the suggestions of his therapist. Has been used as a means to enter occult spirit contact.

Transcendental Meditation—also known as TM, this is a religious pursuit of higher consciousness via meditation as promoted by the followers of the Maharishi Mahesh Yogi.

SV—although touted as a "science" there is little to support the claims of this religious practice which is for all purposes very similar to Hinduism.

SC—a variant of Hinduism which promotes reincarnation, the working out of karma, and salvation based on personal effort through meditation and self-enlightenment.

Yoga—a Hindu philosophical and religious system whose various practices are all used to further one's path toward "union with Brahma."

SV—little evidence for medical effectiveness beyond an improvement of flexibility and relaxation.

SC—a potential entry point for unsuspecting persons seeking improved health to become enmeshed in this Hindu practice designed as a way of personal salvation or way to union with God.

Energy Manipulating Therapies

Acupuncture—a part of traditional Chinese medicine in which needles are placed at specific points believed to treat various ailments and organs often at areas remote to the insertion sites.

SV—a controversial practice with limited clinical use at best. Conflicting reports suggest a strong component of placebo and suggestion involved in acupuncture.

SC—a system of treatment based on the manipulation of an unproven "universal energy" with its basis in Eastern mystical religious philosophy.

Applied Kinesiology—a system of diagnosis and treatment through muscle testing based on the concept of universal energy.

SV—no scientific validity.

SC—promotes the concept of universal energy and monism.

Crystals—mineral rocks said by some to have healing powers.

SV—no scientific evidence.

SC—promotes the concept of universal energy and monism.

Flower Remedies—medicines made by placing flowers in water and exposing it to sunlight.

SV—no validity in basically a homeopathic variation implying the imparting of the flower's spiritual essence to the solution.

SC—another promotion of the universal energy concept.

Iridology—a system of diagnosis and treatment based on the reading of the iris or colored part of your eye.

SV—no validity having failed scientific evaluation on numerous occasions.

SC—practiced alone there is no spiritual danger in this false method, however, often used in conjunction with other universal energy methods.

Reflexology—medical treatment by pressing certain areas of the feet to effect change in remote and unconnected areas of the body.

SV—no validity and anatomically impossible.

SC—mechanism of action is typically a promotion of the universal energy concept.

Reiki—healing methods through manipulation of a person's energy.

SV—no validity and in many cases the patient is not even touched.

SC—promotes the universal energy concept and use of altered consciousness by both patient and healer.

Therapeutic Touch—a variant of other energy manipulating systems typically promoted within the nursing profession.

SV—no consistent scientific evidence.

SC—universal energy concept.

Universal Energy—an unseen force supposedly running through all of creation and the universe which by many is considered to actually be God. It is something which through various methods can supposedly be controlled for good or bad.

SV—no scientific evidence for such a force.

SC—an ancient Eastern metaphysical concept called by different names in different cultures and religions. Energy is a god-
like substance for many Eastern religions such as Hinduism,
Unity, and Taoism.

Supernatural Therapies

Channeling—the action of a person communicating information
from an unseen spirit.

SV—no scientific evidence to support such activities.

SC—a clear violation of Biblical warnings not to consult with
familiar spirits and an open invitation to demonic influence.

Psychic Surgery—removal of diseased parts of the body through
supposedly supernatural means without the usual techniques of surgery and anesthesia.

SV—no validity based on a scientific explanation with numerous cases of documented fraud and deception.

SC—typically coupled with religious symbols and sometimes
performed by so-called "Reverends."

Shamanism—a system of spiritual and medical intervention via a
healer adept in entering altered consciousness to communicate between the physical and the spirit world.

SV—any episodes of healing unexplained by normal physical
means.

SC—direct communication with the spirit world and an opening up for demonic influence by both patients and practitioners.

Spirit Guide—a conjured up entity while in a state of altered consciousness which supposedly gives advice and support to the seeker.

SV—scientifically unproven.

SC—a demonic spirit which may appear in many forms and
typically has an anti-Christian and unbiblical message.

Visualization—an attempt to create your own reality through states
of altered consciousness.

SV—conflicting evidence for beneficial effects other than relaxation.

SC—any technique promoting an altered state of consciousness invites demonic influence especially when coupled with the practice of seeking for a spirit guide.

NOTES

Chapter 1

1. Victor Herbert, M. D., J. D., "Unproven (Questionable) Dietary and Nutritional Methods in Cancer Prevention and Treatment," *Cancer,* 58: 1930–1941, Oct. 15, 1986.
2. Multnomah County Medical Society, "Understanding and Combatting Health Fraud and Quackery," Multnomah County Medical Society, Portland, OR, 1985.
3. Pat Samples, "Different Drummers," *American Medical News,* Aug. 3, 1990, 25.
4. Kristin Olsen, *The Encyclopedia of Alternative Health Care* (New York: Pocket Books, 1989), 16.

Chapter 2

1. Gilda Radner, *It's Always Something* (New York: Simon & Schuster, 1989), 65.
2. Ibid. 66.
3. Herbert, M.D., J.D., "Unproven (Questionable) Dietary and Nutritional Methods."
4. Stephen Barrett, M.D., *Health Schemes, Scams, and Frauds* (New York: Comsumer Reports Books, 1990).
5. Radner, *It's Always Something*, 148.
6. Ibid. 220.
7. Monte Kline, "God's Plan for Your Body," audiotape.
8. Barbara Sigmund, "I Didn't Give Myself Cancer," *CA—A Cancer Journal for Clinicians,* Vol. 40, No. 4, July/August 1990.
9. Richard Leviton, "Who Calls the Shots," *East-West,* Nov. 1988.

Chapter 3

1. Bernie S. Siegel, *Love, Medicine & Miracles* (New York: Harper and Row, 1986), 149.
2. Ibid., 36.
3. Ibid., 19.
4. Ibid., 219.
5. Ibid., 220.

6. Olsen, *The Encyclopedia of Alternative Health Care,* 16.

7. Bob Larson, *Straight Answers on the New Age* (Nashville: Thomas Nelson, 1989).

8. Siegel, *Love, Medicine & Miracles,* 179.

9. Ibid.

10. "Reiki," *New Age Chicago,* 11: 7, Winter, 1981.

11. Alain Sanders, *Time,* July 16, 1990, 52.

12. Elisabeth Kübler-Ross, *Death: The Final Stage of Growth* (Englewood, NJ: Prentice-Hall, 1975), 119.

13. Raymond Moody, *Life After Life* (New York, Bantam, 1976).

14. William Wilson, "Seeing the Light," *Special Report,* Oct.–Dec. 1990, 43–50.

15. Maurice Rawlings, M.D., *Beyond Death's Door* (New York: Benton, 1978), xi.

16. Ibid., xiii.

17. Lennie Kronisch, "Elisabeth Kübler-Ross: Messenger of Love," *Yoga Journal,* Nov.–Dec., 1976, 20.

Chapter 4

1. Randall Baer, *Inside the New Age Nightmare* (Lafayette, LA: Huntington House, 1989), 83.

2. Bill Thomson, "Metaphysicians: M.D.'s with a Spiritual Twist," *East-West,* May 1989.

3. Bernie Siegel, *Peace, Love and Healing* (New York: Harper & Row, 1986), 38.

4. Victor Herbert, *Nutrition Cultism* (New York: George F. Stickly Company, 1980), 83.

5. James Lowell, Ph.D., "Mexican Cancer Clinics," *Dubious Cancer Treatment,* American Cancer Society, 1991, 58.

6. Stephen Barrett, *The Health Robbers* (Philadelphia: George F. Stickley, 1980), 162.

7. Victor Herbert, *Nutrition Cultism: Facts and Fiction* (Philadelphia: George F. Stickley, 1981).

8. John H. Renner, M.D., *HealthSmarts* (Kansas City, MO: HealthFacts, 1990).

9. Stephen Barrett, M.D., and Barrie Cassileth, Ph.D., *Dubious Cancer Treatment* (American Cancer Society, 1991).

10. Baer, *Inside the New Age Nightmare,* 154.

Chapter 5

1. *The Austin American Statesman,* June 25, 1989.

2. Dina Van Pelt, "The Medicine of Mind over Malady," *Insight,* July 16, 1990.

3. *Positive Living and Health* (Emmaus, PA: Rodale Press, 1990), 325.

4. Douglas B. Gates, D.C., Dean of Continuing Education, Sherman College of Chiropractic, in "The Sherman Report," 1975.

5. Mark Sanders, "Take It From a D.C.: A Lot of Chiropractic is a Sham," *Medical Economics,* Sept. 17, 1990.

6. ACA Article, *American Chiropractic Association Journal,* 1989, 37.

7. Catherine Gabe, "Alternative Healthcare," *The Plaindealer Magazine,* Sept. 17, 1989.

8. Oliver Wendell Holmes, "Homeopathy," in *Examining Holistic Medicine,* ed. by Douglas Stalker and Clark Glymour (Buffalo, NY: Prometheus, 1985).

9. Andrew Weil, *Health and Healing* (Boston: Houghton-Mifflin, 1988), 37.

10. "Macrobiotic Diets for the Treatment of Cancer," *CA—A Cancer Journal for Clinicians,* Vol. 39, No. 4, July–August 1989.

11. Mishio Kushi, Kushi Institute literature and promotional materials.

12. Ibid.

13. Ibid.

14. Jonathan Halper, "Naturopaths and Childhood Immunizations: Heterodoxy Among the Unorthodox," *Pediatrics,* Vol. 68, No. 3, September 1981.

Chapter 6

1. Ramona Cass, "We Let Our Son Die," *Journal of Christian Nursing,* Spring 1987, 4–8.

2. Norman Cousins, *Anatomy of an Illness* (New York: Bantam, 1981), 19.

3. H. W. Dresser, *A History of the New Thought Movement* (London: George G. Harrup), 118–119.

4. *Facts About Christian Science* (Boston: The Christian Science Publishing Society, 1959), 5.

5. Ibid., 6.

6. Ibid., 7.

7. Ibid., 10.

8. Frederick Peabody, *The Religo-Medical Masquerade* (Old Tappan, NJ: Revell, 1910), 113.

9. *Children's Healthcare is a Legal Duty,* Child Newsletter, No. 4, 1989.

10. *Facts About Christian Science* (Boston: The Christian Science Publishing Society, 1959), 20.

11. Nathan Talbott, "The Position of the Christian Science Church," *New England Journal of Medicine,* Vol. 309, No. 26, December 29, 1983.

12. Science of Mind literature.

13. Bernie Zilbergeld, Ph.D., et al eds., *Hypnosis: Questions and Answers* (New York: W. W. Norton Company, 1989).

14. Ibid.

15. Ibid., 107.

16. *Dallas Morning News,* February 4, 1990.

17. Maharishi Mahesh Yogi, *Transcendental Meditation* (New York: Signet, 1968), 298–300.

18. Colin Campbell, "Transcendence Is As American As Ralph Waldo Emerson," *Psychology Today,* April 1974, 38.

19. Advertisement for Vedenta Press and Bookshop in *Yoga Journal,* Nov.– Dev. 1989, 34.

Chapter 7

1. Max Mueller, ed., *Sacred Books of the East* (London: Krishna Press), 1879–1910.

2. Ronald Kotzsch, "Acupuncture Today," *East-West,* Jan. 1986, 61.

3. Clive Johnson, "Touch for Health," *Science of Mind,* Sept. 1977, 99.

4. Russell Chandler, *Understanding the New Age* (Dallas: Word Publishing, 1988).

5. Jake Page, "Supreme Quartz," *Omni,* August 1990.

6. Randall Baer, *Inside the New Age Nightmare* (Lafayette, LA: Huntington House, 1989,) 22.

7. Ibid., 36.

8. Ibid., 132.

9. Ibid., 55.

10. *Olsen, The Encyclopedia of Alternate Health Care,* 94.

11. Advertisement for a lecturing iridologist, Joyce Provence, in Phoenix, Arizona.

12. Bernard Jensen, *A New Lifestyle for Health and Happiness* (Escondido, CA: self-published, 1980), 27.

13. Janet Macrae, *Therapeutic Touch: A Practical Guide* (Westminster, NJ: Alfred Knopf, 1987).

14. Bob Larson, *Straight Answers on the New Age* (Nashville: Thomas Nelson, 1990).

Chapter 8

1. Morton Kelsey, *Healing and Christianity* (New York: Harper & Row, 1976), 51.

2. Advertisement for *The Jesus Letters,* in the discount catalog for Lor'd Industries, 52.

3. C. Norman Shealy, M.D., *Occult Medicine Can Save Your Life* (Canal Winchester, OH: Ariel, 1975).

4. Mena, "Conversations with Mena," *Arizona Light,* July 1989, 14.

5. Association for Research and Enlightenment membership promotional literature.

6. W. Rice, "A Surgeon's Magic Touch That's Too Good To Be True," *Today's Health,* June 1974, 54–59.

7. Michael Harner, *A Guide to Power and Healing: The Way of the Shaman* (New York: Barton, 1980), xiii.

8. Ibid., 175.

9. Gerald Epstein, M.D., *Healing Visualizations: Creating Health Through Imagery* (New York: Bantam, 1989), copyright.

10. Ibid., 39.

11. Ibid., 54–55.

Chapter 9

1. In his article in *The New Zealand Medical Journal,* August 9, 1989.

2. James Goodwin, "The Tomato Effect: Rejection of Highly Efficacious Therapies," *The Journal of the American Medical Association,* May 11, 1981.

3. Marian Segal, "Defrauding the Desperate: Quackery and AIDS," *FDA Consumer,* Oct. 1987.

4. Elizabeth Gettig, "Faith Healing: A Case Presentation," *Birth Defects,* Vol. 23, No. 6, 1987.

5. James Randi, *The Faith Healers* (Buffalo, NY: Prometheus Books, 1987), 298.

6. Hank Hanegraff, "Faith in Faith or Faith in God?" *The Christian Research Institute Journal,* Winter/Spring 1990.

Chapter 10

1. Maurice Smith, "Guidelines for Assessing Iridology and Similar Alternative Health Care Techniques," Home Mission Board, Southern Baptist Convention, 1989.

2. *Newsweek* Gallup Poll, 1989 and National Opinion Research Council of the University of Chicago, 1988.

3. Michael Harner, *A Guide to Power and Healing: The Way of the Shaman* (New York: Barton, 1980), 176–178.

4. Brooks Alexander, "The Sellout of Science," *Spiritual Counterfeits Project Journal,* August 1978, 22.

5. Johnny M. Lamb, "The Shamanic Side of Surgery," *Military Medicine,* Vol. 153, Oct. 1988, 541.

6. Mimi Swartz, "The Ornish Treatment," *Texas Monthly,* March 1991.